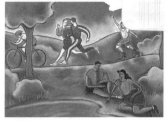

Inspired

to

Lose

Motivational Stories
From
North America's Leading
Weight-Loss Support Group

Howard J. Rankin, Ph.D

Published by StepWise Press
Hilton Head Island, South Carolina

First printing, June, 2001

Copyright © Howard J. Rankin
All rights reserved

Library of Congress Catalog Card Number 2001117651
ISBN: 0-9658261-4-7

Printed in the United States

CONTENTS

Acknowledgements

Both new friends and old acquaintances helped with this project. In some cases, the project has turned old acquaintances into new friends and names on a file into rewarding and uplifting relationships.

My first acknowledgement is to the many TOPS members who submitted stories. Their enthusiasm and goodwill made the project not only possible but also exciting, an adventure that every day produced new revelations. I salute the contributors whose stories appear here. Everyone was not only willing to share his personal story but did so primarily in the hope that it would help others.

I also want to thank the TOPS Board of Directors for supporting the project. So heartfelt thanks to Betty Domenoe, Gina Brueske, Barbara Cady, LaNeida Herrick, Jeanne Myatt, Jean Terpstra, Imogene Welch, Shirley Wooten, and especially Nancy Best, the Board's liaison on this project, who supported the concept so wholeheartedly.

Gail Schemberger, TOPS Headquarters Director, and Susan Trones, TOPS Communications Director, also were unstinting in their support and help with research. Many others at, or associated with, TOPS helped, including Ken Donner and Bea Miller.

This project may never have gotten off the ground if it were not for the insight, enthusiasm, support, and sheer professionalism of Celia Rocks. Celia and the company Rocks-DeHart had been recommended to me as book consultants with a great reputation. That reputation is well earned and more than justified. When *Inspired to Lose* was merely a concept, Celia was able to fashion the notion and sculpt it into a book that I believe really will inspire and help people manage their weight and their health. Celia's associates, Ann Keller and Dottie DeHart, also contributed significantly to the project.

Finally, special thanks and much love go to family who have watched the gestation of this project with as much enthusiasm as I have. My wife, M. J., has been a great supporter and also offered some timely insights. James has endured my long hours spent away at the computer with good humor and grace, as has Josh. Ellen, as always, has been a constant support and a delightful presence.

Introduction

Successful weight loss is more than pounds lost. Successful weight loss is about self-esteem, identity, hope, and self-affirmation. For many people, weight loss is merely symptomatic of deeper, personal change.

I have learned these things in a twenty-five year career in which I have researched and treated weight problems from several different viewpoints. As a scientist at the University of London's Addiction Research Unit, I spent ten years examining the nature of addiction and exploring ways of defusing compulsive behaviors, including weight-control issues.

One study looked at the role of family support in weight-loss efforts. A different study, conducted in 1975, focused on the psychology of sensible weight loss and was written up in the popular press as the "no-diet diet." Other research addressed the perception of portion size. In this study, women were asked to rate the taste of several foods and were told that they could eat as much of the foods as they wished in order to make their ratings. Subjects were then asked to estimate how much they had eaten, and this was compared to actual amounts. All subjects knew the calorie values of the foods very well, but the actual amounts eaten were significantly underestimated.

When I became disenchanted with the academic life, I moved to St. Andrews Hospital, a nonprofit hospital in Northampton where I ran the Eating Disorders Unit and discovered that weight, eating, and body-image are lethal weapons that can be used destructively against others or oneself.

I was recruited to America in 1986 for a position as clinical director of a private behavioral medicine program that focused on weight loss. I observed first hand the constant struggle against obesity. During my tenure as clinical director I met many interesting and wonderful people, clients and colleagues alike. One of these was Dr. Ahmed Kissebah, one of the world's leading obesity geneticists and Chief of the Department of Endocrinology, Metabolism and Clinical Nutrition at the Medical College of Wisconsin. It was Ahmed who created the waist-hip ratio as a useful and reliable measure of disease risk, and it was he who introduced me to the nonprofit weight-loss support group, Take Off Pounds Sensibly, or TOPS.

After nine years as clinical director it was time for me to move on and explore a developing area of psychology of monumental importance—the relationship between mind and body.

Research in mind-body medicine shows quite conclusively that the mind and body are not separate entities but are also interconnected and interchangeable. Many aspects of this incredible cellular network are not just mind-boggling (or even mind-body-boggling) but also crucial in understanding health and behavior. I am fascinated by the fact that different memories are held in various parts of the body and by the idea—according to the discoverer of the brain's endorphin receptors, Candace Pert—that your body *is* your subconscious. There is no doubt in my mind that the physical self is a reflection of the psychological and spiritual self.

Your body is your subconscious.

Another critical aspect of mind-body research focuses on the healing power of positive relationships, a central theme of this book. Human beings are social animals and, like other social species, physical and emotional contact is essential for well-being and optimum functioning. To pick just one example of many available, the work of Dean Ornish is particularly illustrative. Ornish, a cardiologist and lifestyle change expert, has reached the conclusion that relationships are the most powerful element in healing those with heart disease. His book,

Love and Survival, describes a mass of evidence supporting the notion that meaningful contact with others is a fundamental part of healing. Psychological repair goes hand-in-hand with physical repair. Psychological healing is not only a consequence of physical healing, but also a cause of it.

It was while in the midst of grappling with these themes that Ahmed approached me to cooperate in the writing of a new guidebook for TOPS. He is TOPS' Medical Advisor and, with some of that group's financial support and an enormous and heroic effort by their volunteer members, he has completed the most significant study on the genetics of obesity that has been, or is ever likely to be, conducted. Details of that ongoing story are available at the Health Professionals/Research section of the TOPS website: www.tops.org.

After I cowrote the TOPS guidebook, *The Choice Is Yours*, I became more involved in the organization. I was soon won over by the charm and grace of many of the people involved in it. I was impressed with the simplicity of the organization's message and the importance of its mission. Here are thousands of people whose goal is simply to help one another battle the most serious public health issue of our time. Almost exclusively there is little or no financial reward. The only reason people are involved in TOPS, from the board down to the ordinary members, is that they care.

As I traveled the country attending TOPS meetings, I met more of the organization's nearly quarter of a million members and heard some incredible stories of courage, passion, commitment, and purpose. These stories reinforced and informed my own views, not just on the process of weight loss but also on personal transformation in general. Here were stories that needed to be told.

TOPS is about the incredible healing power of positive group and personal interaction. I could have filled volumes with literally thousands of stories of people, desperate to lose weight, who were at the end of the line physically and emotionally but found within TOPS the loving care and practical support that inspired them to change their lives.

Some of those stories do appear here, but in the interest of balanced and diversified communication, I have included stories of various shapes, colors, and textures that inspire and support at different levels. So in this book you will find everything from complete life histories—big picture inspiration—to short one-page vignettes that will give you insight on single but significant weight-loss behaviors.

All of the stories are from TOPS members. Some of the stories specifically focus on the TOPS experience; others do not. Every person who submitted a piece for consideration for this book, without exception, did so because she wanted to give back, not just to the organization but to anyone who needed help. These are people who know what it is like to battle one's weight and what is needed to succeed.

The Weight of the World

Nowhere is personal transformation more evident than in, or more sought after than by, the overweight. In a competitive and materialist society, excess weight can mean failure. In a society that often fails to distinguish between striving for perfection and achieving it, we have the concept of ideal weight that is almost impossible to maintain. In a society that is only interested in results rather than process, buttock measurements are the bottom line. These trends pressure the vast majority of women and a sizable minority of men to spend significant resources trying to control their weight.

Much is known about obesity. We know that modern life only exaggerates the natural trend of the body to gain weight once we get past the ripe old age of thirty-five. To maintain early adult weight, calorie intake needs to be reduced. Emerging technology, however, allows us to be more sedentary and to get more done by moving less. Computer chips have turned us into couch potatoes. Not only do we know why people gain weight, but we also know what to do about it. Yet most are depressingly unsuccessful at putting these straightforward, corrective behaviors into practice.

In my previous position as a clinical director responsible for seminars on weight loss, I gave the opening presentation for the two-week program to people who had paid a significant amount of money to participate.

"Want to know how to lose weight?" I started. "Eat less fat and exercise. Two thousand dollars, please."

Despite knowing what to do to lose weight, most cannot—for some reason—manage to do it with any consistency. In response to this conundrum, the vast majority search for the Holy Grail in the form of supplements, pills, and fad diets. This external search is fruitless because the answer does not exist outside of our own selves. As you will read in Chapter Five, this search for the Holy Grail is not just fruitless, but it is also sometimes lethal. Any bullet—even a magic one—can be deadly.

The answer does not exist outside but is utterly and completely within us. As these stories show, the real challenge to transformation is not about what to do but *about having the courage and desire to really do it.*

The answer does not exist outside but is utterly and completely within us.

Weight Loss—A Journey Not a Destination

There is an information overload on diet and exercise. Nutritional trends, exercise gimmicks, and dietary fads grab the headlines. This emphasis on the tangible actions necessary for weight management misses the point. It puts the cart before the horse because it assumes that knowledge of what to do is the critical element in weight control. It is not. Most people know what they should be doing to manage their lives, including their weight, but there is a vast gap between knowledge and action.

It is easy in a materialist society to value only the tangible. In so many ways we lose touch with the symbolic value of our actions and fail to acknowledge the real meaning of our behavior. The wrong emphasis in weight loss has made weight loss per se a goal. As you will read in this book, people don't embark on weight-loss programs to lose pounds; they embark on such programs to change their lives. They lose weight to raise self-esteem and create a better self.

A Career in Obesity?

When I was researching and treating addictions in London in the 1970s, my boss was a brilliant and delightful man named Griffith Edwards. Professor Edwards was one of the world's leading addictionologists, and he developed the concept of the natural history of addiction. His idea was that addicts really had a career in addictions. Their addictions were interwoven with the developmental stages of their lives, and many addicts moved in and out of use and abuse of drugs. The same can be easily seen with obesity. As you read these stories you will find that many people moved in and out of obesity, their condition and its management swayed by the winds of maturity and life circumstances. As a result, weight loss is not an end point. Reaching a goal weight is not a final destination but a milestone on life's journey.

Weight can and does fluctuate widely, leading many people to morbid obesity. There are several people featured in this book who have lost more than a hundred pounds and even some who have lost twice that amount and kept it off. Ten years ago, I would have thought twice about including stories of such heavy people for fear that they were so distant from everyday reality that few people could identify with them. That is not the case today. Currently more than 60 percent of the population is officially classified as overweight and millions more as obese and morbidly obese.

While the health challenges of morbid obesity are typically more severe than for the less obese, the same weight-loss tactics and strategies work for everyone. The fact that the strategies worked for the morbidly obese individuals is testimony to their power. It doesn't matter whether you have forty pounds or 240 pounds to lose, the psychology of weight and weight loss remains the same.

Prejudice—A Majority Discrimination

One of the themes that runs through many of the stories is the pervasive prejudice that exists against overweight people. It begins with the cruel ostracism and isolation in the schoolyard and continues through life. Within these stories you will find incidents of children being traumatized not just by other children, but also by teachers and an educational system that at one time thought public humiliation was good motivation. You will read about incidents of bias and brutal treatment by "friends," family, coworkers, superiors, and even complete strangers who reach into shopping carts and remove items they judge inappropriate for an overweight person to buy.

Prejudice and bias are based on fear. In the case of prejudice against the overweight, the prejudiced person's fear might be of losing control, of being overweight himself, or of being socially isolated. Prejudice exists and continues despite the increase in the fat population. Ironically, given that well over half the population is overweight, such prejudice is the first example of *majority* discrimination.

In my conversations, feelings about weight within families presented a more complex picture. Spouses could be unbelievably supportive, openly critical, sneakily sabotaging, or totally indifferent. Children, however, were another matter. Unanimously, overweight parents imagined that their children were embarrassed and ashamed of them. Almost unanimously, children told those same parents, often later in life, that they felt no such humiliation and that it did not influence their love for or their relationship with them one iota.

Perhaps children don't want to hurt their parents by admitting their embarrassment, and this is probably true in some cases. In the case of many to whom I talked, however, these discussions with children took place when the parents were no longer overweight and when an offspring's admission of embarrassment would have been far less hurtful.

The obvious conclusion is that physical appearance is very low down on the list of factors that influence a child's relationship with her parents, but very high up that list in less-intimate relationships. The one exception to that rule might be spouses.

The dialogue we have with others is a reflection of the dialogue we have with ourselves. Many obese women are ashamed and embarrassed about their appearance, and their self-esteem sinks as low as a limbo dancer on Xanax. This projection of self-deprecation has many consequences on daily life that can affect a spouse, especially in the area of intimacy. The devastating effects of obesity on self-esteem are highlighted in Chapter Two where you will find stories of truly remarkable transformations.

It's Always Something

As a psychologist, I talk to people for a living. People talk to me about the meaning or lack thereof in their lives, about the joys and the traumas and the events that fashion their existence. Talking to the people whose stories are featured in this book was no exception. As a result these pages are filled with the realities of life. Some of these stories may read like soap operas, but I guarantee you that they are typical of everyday life. Love, loss, trauma, conflict are part of everyone's life. As Gilda Radner used to say, "It's always something." And we all have something.

In therapy, it is a well-known phenomenon that the client reveals some of the most important details just as the session is about to end. Sometimes that is a matter of trust, sometimes a breakdown of the client's inhibition, sometimes the desire of the client to get his money's worth. Generally, people who submitted stories were extraordinarily patient in dealing with my questions and often very forthcoming about details of their private lives. Occasionally, I would get a nugget of information that was almost a throwaway comment as I was finalizing a story which may not have seemed important to the storyteller but was critical to me. Universally, those who submitted stories were willing to share personal details in the hope that it would help others.

The Power of Others

No man is an island, and those who aspire to be are more Alcatraz than Hilton Head. As I describe in my book, Power Talk: The Art of Effective Communication, social proof is one of the seven fundamental motivators of human action. As much as we like to view ourselves as rugged individualists, the truth is that we depend greatly on the behavior of others to guide and validate our actions.

Given the enormous power of social influence, it is no surprise that each of the people featured in this book required the structured social support of a group like TOPS. Transformation requires not just motivation and skills but also social support. Few, if any, can effect meaningful change on their own. The metamorphosing caterpillar requires the right conditions to complete its transformation into a butterfly. Humans need the right conditions, too. Whereas the caterpillar needs the right temperature, sufficient light, and adequate moisture, human beings require other people to effect their transformation.

There are many ways in which others exert positive influence on our lives. Professor Randy Black of Purdue University has identified four types of support: informing, encouraging, facilitating, and anchoring. Of these, the latter may be the most important and the most difficult to find. Anchoring refers to the technique of providing perspective and positive support for another, especially when that person is having a difficult time and is in danger of relapsing. In every one of the stories contained in this book, there were times when the featured person was struggling to maintain her effort and was full of doubt that she would ever be successful. On each occasion, someone else guided her out of the dark shadows of her doubt.

How people exert their influence seems almost random. Chance comments can ignite profound effects, whereas more direct approaches can fizzle. I believe that indirect approaches are often more powerful because most of us want to feel that we are in control. Reaching a conclusion ourselves is much more powerful precisely because it is our discovery, and as a result we are much more likely not just to accept the message but also to really *own* it. In many of the cases cited in this book, others' comments were influential because they resonated with heretofore-unappreciated inner voices. As many of the cases here also show, timing is everything. Catching a person at the precise moment when he is vulnerable but not defensive seems to be critical in delivering influential messages.

Uncertainty

One of the overriding themes of this book is that we never know what life events mean at the time that we are experiencing them. As the Scandinavian philosopher Kierkegaard said, "Life is best understood backward but has to be lived forward." The clear message from these stories is that we can, with conscious effort, turn a crisis into an opportunity. If we are aware of the possibility and are prepared to act with courage, faith, and commitment, then almost anything can have positive value and meaning. During the darkest times, we need to recognize that the meaning of the events that currently torment us is unknown and that there can be a silver lining in even the blackest of clouds. We need faith to believe that a traumatic event has value even if it is currently impossible to imagine what that value might be.

In the movie, *Apollo 13*, there is a scene in which recorded interviews with the astronauts are being broadcast as the world waits anxiously for news of the astronauts' return to Earth. An interviewer asks Commander Jim Lovell about coping with danger. Lovell describes an incident during World War II in which he was faced with trying to land his damaged plane on the aircraft carrier, the Shangri-La, in the Sea of Japan, despite the fact that his radar was out, the carrier had no running lights, and his homing device was jammed. He was completely lost without any sense of where the carrier was. Just when he thought it couldn't get any worse, it did.

"I switched on my cockpit lights and zap—everything shorted out. I had no lights, I had no instruments—I didn't even know what altitude I was flying at. I was thinking of ditching the plane right there in that vast dark ocean. I looked down, and there in the black ocean was a green carpet—it was algae, the phosphorescent stuff that is churned up in the wake of a big ship—and it was leading me home. Now, if I hadn't turned on my cockpit lights and all my power shorted out there was no way I would ever have seen that. So you never know, you never know, what events are going to transpire to lead you home."

The people featured in this book had no idea that the events in their lives were leading them home. Many of them surely felt that these events were leading them to destruction, misery, and death. With openness, conscious choices, and the help of others, however, they managed to use their circumstances to transform themselves. They needed a kick-start, however, with emphasis on the kick.

Motivation, Motivation, Motivation

I am fascinated by what motivates us to change our lives. I am interested in why we can be motivated by the words of one person when the exact words from someone else make us resist even more. I want to know why Joan can be motivated by an event, and Jane can be discouraged by it.

In these pages you will read about different motivators, and you will learn about stages of change. Some of the people were motivated by seemingly trivial events, others by significant traumas. In general, however, motivation stems from discomfort caused by the contradiction between what we believe and how we behave.

Part of the motivation puzzle has already been solved. Twenty years ago psychologists Jim Prochaska and Carlo DiClemente gave us a model of motivation that suggested people move through different stages on their way to positive action and transformation. Subsequent research and clinical intuition tells us what helps people move through those motivational stages. Typically, change begins when we are forced to face up to the inconsistency in our morals, values, and behaviors. Some of us need nudging out of the denial that characterizes this inconsistency, some need blasting out, and some are simply incapable of ever venturing beyond their comfortable blindness.

Having motivation and maintaining it are two different propositions. Motivation ebbs and flows like the tide, and there is the real danger that at the precise moment when we need to stay afloat and keep buoyant, the tide will be out and we will be marooned in the mud of our own helplessness. Capturing motivation so that it can be called on in time of need is as important as finding it in the first place.

Successful people find ways of keeping their motivation in the forefront of their minds. All of the individuals featured in this book found their own way of maintaining motivation. No matter how individually colored the process may be, it always comes down to finding some way of keeping in touch with the real meaning of the struggle. So whether it is a phrase, a rhyme, a photo, or some other token, successful people not only keep their eyes on the prize but also remain connected to the symbolic meaning of achieving it.

Successful people find ways of keeping their motivation in the forefront of their minds.

Relationships and Health

I am convinced that the key to health, life, and happiness is the quality of relationships. There is so much evidence showing the necessity of good relationships for health and well-being that it is surprising that there has not been more emphasis on group support for all areas of health. But, if we need research to tell us that connections with others are critical, then we are in bad shape. Human beings are social animals, and it is important to recognize that meaningful social contact, especially in an increasingly isolating world, is essential.

It does take a village to raise a child, and it takes a community to raise adults. We have lost the enormous value of community—the trust, the support, and the caring of family; the structure of the tribe; and the wisdom of elders. Psychologists and mental-health professionals have proliferated to take the place of these fundamental family and community supports and, frankly, we'd be better off with the original system.

The original system has long since passed, though. Finding others who can identify with problems, provide honest feedback, give valuable information, and do so in complete trust and confidence is no easy feat. Where people can be brought together in such a way, the effects can be overwhelmingly powerful. There is no more potent force for personal empowerment than a good group.

There is no more potent force for personal empowerment than a good group.

TOPS and Weight-Loss Support

Group weight-loss support does not just have to come from TOPS. It's just that TOPS happens to be the group I know, and it is the largest, most established organization of its kind. I do believe it is important, however, that TOPS is a nonprofit organization focusing solely on support. While most commercial organizations offer good services and products, I believe it is difficult for them to maintain a healthy balance between competing goals. How does an organization balance its stated goal to sell its customers products and services with the goal of providing independent support and advice? When weekly dues and counselor fees are part of the program, will such an organization be happy to promote the out-of-session relationships and activities between members that are an essential part of a group like TOPS?

Some commercial groups do a good job in helping people lose weight, but they are not primarily weight-loss *support groups*. TOPS has been around for over fifty years, has almost a quarter of a million members in more than ten thousand chapters, and has a *single* mission to provide weight-loss support. Overeaters Anonymous, which also helps many people, is a support group for *compulsive eating, not weight loss per se*. Which is why I consider TOPS to be America's leading weight-loss support group.

Individual needs vary, and at any one time a person may require the emphasis provided by one organization or another. Moreover, commercial and nonprofit organizations are not mutually exclusive. I do believe that no matter how you are trying to lose weight, the support of others is essential, wherever it is found.

The stories that you are about to read are as much about personal transformation and change as they are about weight loss. If weight is an issue for you, these stories will be especially meaningful. Even if weight is not an issue, however, you will find within these pages valuable lessons about courage, passion, purpose, persistence, and many other qualities that make for a life of fulfillment. I guarantee that you will identify with these stories and that they will help you find your own peace and happiness. All you need is an open mind, a box of tissues, and a highlighter pen. Not only will you find inspiration that can help you, but you will also learn much about how to help others.

Howard J. Rankin, Ph.D
Hilton Head Island
April 2001

Chapter 1

Elements of a Group That Works

Each of the people whose stories are featured in this book regularly attended TOPS groups. Rather than repeat mentioning that experience in each story, I will provide a brief overview of a TOPS meeting and touch upon those elements that I believe, from both clinical experience and the report of members, are the significant elements of weight change.

There are over ten thousand TOPS groups that meet on a weekly basis, each colored by the individuals that make up the groups, so that in some ways there are no typical groups. Some groups have just a few members; others have more than a hundred. Regional, cultural, and individual differences also prevail. There are, however, elements common to each of these groups that are powerful change agents.

Each group begins with a weigh-in. There is a formal position of weight recorder within each group, and this person is responsible for personally weighing and recording each member's weekly weight. Weighing is done individually with the weight recorder present. Weight recorders are sympathetic and encouraging people who know how to share the enthusiasm of a weight loss and moderate the disappointment of a weight gain. The weight recorder is an important position because this person helps members keep their perspective about weight and weight loss.

Fat loss does not equal weight loss. When fat is burned, it takes a while before it can be converted to water and excreted; so it is very possible to have eaten, exercised sensibly, and burned fat but not have that reflected on the scale. Keeping a proper perspective about the scale is essential, and weight recorders are able to do just that. The focus needs to be on behavior—doing the right things—not on what the scale happens to record on any particular week.

Weighing-in is critical because it provides accountability. This is crucial. Without public accountability, it is only human for individuals to lose their focus and quickly lose motivation when struggling with their program. Going public is a prime way to maintain motivation and stay on track.

After weigh-in, the group members will then gather together and individually report their progress for the week. Success is greeted with encouragement, and setbacks are greeted with genuine support and an analysis of how behavior can be changed in the upcoming week. This time, therefore, involves not just support but also practical ways of approaching the week ahead. This is the time, too, when members might offer each other some physical support for the upcoming week. Perhaps arrangements will be made to exercise together or help out in other ways if a member is experiencing difficulties. This help could be anything from offers to provide transport to caring for a sick family member.

Following the roundtable discussion of personal performance, there will then be a presentation on some aspect relevant to weight loss. Members take turns to present material that they have discovered themselves or that is provided to them by TOPS headquarters. The TOPS organization provides literally dozens of programs on subjects related to nutrition, exercise, stress and time management, and many other relevant topics. This part of the program provides not just informational support, but also allows members to share what has worked for them. TOPS supports the Exchange System for guiding food choices. The Exchange System provides nutritional equivalents across food groups.[1]

Groups may then participate in some creative activity, designed to reinforce group cohesion and emphasize weight-loss messages. There might also be contests in which very small amounts of money are put into a kitty and given to those who performed best during the previous week. Small-change fines (typically a quarter or so) might also be levied against participating members for not following through on promised behavioral tasks (e.g., not keeping a proper food diary).

There is a tremendous amount of contact between members outside of meetings. These friendships are essential. Many of the stories in this book show how friendships born out of the TOPS group were critical to ultimate success. People who are dealing with the same issues make good friends, so that the strength of many of the relationships born from TOPS is no surprise. These friendships often transcend weight loss, and the members concerned became lifelong supporters and soul mates.

Accountability, information, support, and friendship—these are the common themes that emerge as the critical elements of the TOPS experience and are powerful vehicles of personal transformation.

Developing Personal Power

Make the right choices; gain control

Destiny is not a matter of chance. It is a matter of choice: it is not a thing to be waited for, it is a thing to be achieved. –
William Jennings Bryan

We control our lives. It is easy to lose sight of this simple fact. Many people never appreciate their power, and it remains dormant and untapped. Others are aware of it, but over time they concede it, giving away their most valuable asset.

There are various reasons for this power failure. Some people are trained to be powerless. These trainers can be family, the culture, or the cruel hand of fate. Ultimately, however, none of these influences can be significant without the consent of the individual who, consciously or otherwise, agrees to forfeit control.

One of the reasons why people concede their power is that they are confused about the difference between control and success. It is tempting to conclude that if success is not forthcoming, any action is futile. That idea assumes that success is an all-or-nothing proposition. It is not.

There are always solutions to problems, but there are not always wonderful solutions. Even if we can't see how to get what we want, there are always plans of action. They may not immediately lead us to the ultimate destination, but that is no reason to retreat into helplessness. Success generally takes time and is generally achieved step by step. Unrealistic views of what constitutes success and the time it takes to reach goals are among the main reasons why so many people fail at weight loss and lifestyle change. They try to make many drastic changes all at once, get frustrated, and give up when this proves too difficult. As many stories in this book demonstrate, starting with small changes and building from there is ultimately a successful strategy.

Many life situations are more about damage control than accomplishment. But damage control is less glamorous than achievement. Damage control also implies limitations that are often uncomfortable to acknowledge. As a result, such limitations, like obesity, are overlooked until they can be overlooked no more.

People also concede power when they are overwhelmed by events. Sometimes life throws a curve ball that seems unhittable. I once had a client who, within the space of three weeks, lost her husband, her father, and her grandfather; watched her son undergo emergency brain surgery; and discovered a key employee had been embezzling, pushing her business to the wall. Yes, she did suffer a meltdown that reduced her to almost catatonic helplessness. This was temporary, however, and she was soon back in the saddle, taking what steps she could to regain control. As she said to me, "I have two choices. I can just sit and do nothing or I can use every resource I have to reclaim my life." Once these words were out of her mouth, the number of choices was reduced to one.

Few people are confronted with the prospect of being swept away on such a tidal wave of misfortune. Instead, most of us face occasional high tides of adversity that can gradually erode our ability to cope and can grind away at hope. At that point there is the real danger of giving up. Be warned, however: Fatalism can be fatal.

History can also be harmful, eroding personal power on the jagged rocks of failure. So many people have a glittering record of failure when it comes to weight loss that to embark on yet another attempt is really the triumph of hope over experience. As pointed out in Chapter Five on responsibility, however, it is not the next diet or any diet that is going to work. The only thing that can work is you.

***It is not the next diet or any diet that is going to work. The
only thing that can work is you.***

Success depends entirely on the acceptance that responsibility rests
within you and you alone. Nevertheless, a history of failure inevitably
leads to resigned acceptance that there is little that can be done. In one
of the stories that follows, Roe WiersGalla had already made up her
mind that she was going to die at 365 pounds and that there was little
she could do about it.

> *What lies behind us and what lies before us are tiny matters*
> *compared to what lies within us.*
> *– Ralph Waldo Emerson*

Whenever I come across individuals whose records of failure have
worn away their hope, I remind them that we do not have to be trapped
by our history. Our past is a teacher, not a jailer. We are free to choose
our destiny, our hands on the tiller today plotting a course to tomorrow. It doesn't matter if you have lost and gained weight a hundred
times; today always presents different possibilities.

If adversity and history can lead to personal power outages, so can
the culture. Taking control of your life means putting yourself first, at
least some of the time. Despite the advances made by women in the
past fifty years, the perception still exists that women are society's nur-
turers and caretakers. That is because they are. Psychologically and bio-
logically women have the capacity to take care of others in a way that
men do not. This is, of course, not the *only* female capacity. They have
many other natural talents and abilities, and the lack of recognition of
these other skills has led some women to a misplaced rejection of their
nurturing nature. The problem is not in the female ability to nurture
but in finding a balance between nurturing and other activities and
between nurturing oneself as well as nurturing others.

Putting oneself first is a necessity for good lifestyle and health practices. I have seen many women whose lifestyle- and health-management efforts have been impaled on the misplaced sword of guilt. They can't seem to overcome the cultural imperatives of taking care of everyone else and so leave themselves at the bottom of the heap.

Learning to define personal boundaries is the key to maintaining power. Draw those boundaries too tight, and nobody can enter your space—leaving you aloof and isolated. Draw those boundaries too wide, and everyone can intrude—draining time, energy, and power.

There are people who will drain your power even if they don't try to steal it from you directly. In my seminars on this topic, I ask members of the audience to make a list of those people in their lives who enhance their weight-control efforts and those who don't. There are many forms of opposition: criticism, negativity, doubt, and open sabotage. On one occasion, I asked the seminar participants to talk about which people were on their respective lists of helpers and saboteurs. One girl admitted, "There is one person who appears on my list as a critic, doubter, saboteur, and negative influence. It's me."

If you pull the plug on your personal power, you are in deep trouble. The only way to keep switched on in times of crisis is to ensure that you are connected to the positive energy of other people. They are your power source.

Taking Action

Twenty years ago, two psychologists, Jim Prochaska and Carlo DiClemente, proposed a five-stage model of motivation. These stages are really different levels of taking action and control. This model speaks eloquently not just to weight management but also to any behavior change. The five stages are as follows: Pre-Contemplation, Contemplation, Preparation, Action, and Maintenance.

Pre-Contemplation is when, through either ignorance or denial, no attention is given to the problem. One of the reasons why problems are avoided is because admitting them has serious repercussions for many other areas of life. For example, recognizing the need to lose weight might also mean recognizing an unhappy marriage, financial uncertainty, or social anxiety. The subconscious miraculously takes all of these factors into account, allowing them to surface only when conscious consideration *could* lead to positive action.

Contemplation is the stage at which there is recognition of the need to take action, but it is not forthcoming. Such contemplation can occur because there are too many difficult implications of following through with action or because the person is not entirely ready.

Preparation is the stage at which the person readies himself for action. In weight management, this might be manifested as getting the phone number of a support group or buying relevant books.

The fourth stage, **Action**, is where positive steps are taken to address the issue. The final stage, **Maintenance**, is where actions are taken to continue the positive steps already taken.

Initially, it was believed that people moved steadily through these stages in turn, but that is not the case. As you can tell from the stories in this book, people move in and out of these stages at different times. In fact, many people go from maintenance back to pre-contemplation in their weight-control efforts.

What is particularly helpful is an understanding of what moves people forward through these stages. Several people featured in this book needed a traumatic event to push them out of helplessness and from pre-contemplation into action. Others are triggered by seemingly more trivial events that are nonetheless just as meaningful to those experiencing them. In virtually every story in this book, what moved people to action was pain. To quote C. S. Lewis, "Pain is God's megaphone." For those who are in the coma of denial and pre-contemplation, God has to shout very loudly through His megaphone to get attention. This means that it is only a BIG PAIN that will initiate action. By the time you get a big pain, however, it may be too late, and there may be nothing you can do. If you are not comatose and comfortably asleep in pre-contemplation but are more aware and open to the idea of change, God doesn't have to shout so loudly to get your attention.

Life *is* what happens when you have other things planned. You can hide; you can run; you can stand and fight. But whatever you do, there will be consequences. Even if you do nothing, there are consequences. There is no such thing as doing *nothing*. Inactivity is a choice. Helplessness is a state of mind, not a reality.

Events, history, culture, and other people can threaten to overwhelm us. In the end, however, we are the only ones who can take away our power. Our power is surrendered *by* us, not taken *from* us.

In the stories that follow you will be reminded that every action is a choice and that every choice has a price and a payoff. In the end, facing up to significant issues is the only choice. You just have to make sure that you don't leave your positive choices too late.

The Server Changed—Betsy Lavin

Betsy Lavin's story is about a determined woman who finally was able to move beyond guilt and obligation and find the meaning of her life and thus her health.

Betsy Lavin's story is all about choice. Hers is a story that speaks to the heart of every woman. Unlike several other stories featured in this book, Betsy was not overweight as a child, and her excess weight did not cause major health problems. Betsy's story is typical in that it speaks to the very core of a fundamental female question — when is the woman's tremendous capacity for care taking and caring applied to herself rather than others?

Betsy grew up in rural America, a double-edged sword from a health perspective. On the one hand, there was always lots of meat, potatoes, and home-style cooking with unlimited supplies of whole milk, cheese, and ice cream around. On the other hand, there was a farm on which to roam, play, and work. Consumed calories were burned when doing chores. Betsy's mother was a great believer in chiropractic medicine and would regularly take Betsy and her sister to the local chiropractor, not just for skeletal adjustments but also to treat all manner of other, mild health problems.

So Betsy grew up totally unconcerned or occupied with weight. It was not until she was in her late twenties that she was aware of weight being a problem. But when she was fifteen her weight did increase significantly—she was pregnant.

"There was never ever any question that I wouldn't keep the child," says Betsy, who gave birth to Chad in July 1978. A few months later she was married to Chad's dad and a junior in high school. Becoming a mother did create some changes. For one thing, she had to quit sports at which she excelled. She did gain some weight during pregnancy, but eventually that came off. Betsy accepted the responsibility of her new role with youthful ignorance. This was going to be like it was supposed to be: be married, have a family, take care of husband and children, and live happily ever after.

There were a couple of other girls in Betsy's school that were in the same predicament. And predicament is how most people perceived being a married mother two years away from high school graduation.

"We were seen as different. Times were changing, however. Twenty years earlier we would have been outcasts. At least the school made some attempt to help us with stuff like prenatal classes that were held in the school library. Still, the general consensus from the community was, 'What a shame. Any potential is wasted. What can you amount to now?'" says Betsy.

Betsy definitely sensed the negativity from some of the small community members but tried not to let the stereotype deflect her from her studies. Following her pregnancy she had given up whatever hope she had of ever going to college, but she worked diligently to get good grades in some of the less-demanding courses. There was no point in taking math and science courses if she wasn't going to college, she figured.

The stereotyping of her made Betsy sensitive to what other people thought about her. Sensitive maybe, but determined to take charge of her life.

"I truly knew that God had more in store for me than just being a mom and a housewife," says Betsy.

Some changes happened quickly. Soon after she graduated from high school she was divorced. Now she was faced with finding a job and raising her son. Within two months she had moved to the Twin Cities.

Betsy tried several jobs. She sold vacuum cleaners. She sold vacuum cleaners so well that she won all sorts of awards. Before long she had her own small business, but this failed because of youthful inexperience.

She had a job at a stockbroker's but realized that this wasn't for her. She sold and modeled clothes at in-home parties but realized that this wasn't for her either. She was a waitress. She was a very good waitress at some of the finest restaurants, but that wasn't her life's calling either.

Now the financial pressures and other obligations of being a single mom in her late twenties were really beginning to hit home. Betsy became desperate. She realized it was time for a change.

She decided to become a chiropractor.

She did not have the scientific qualifications. She did not have more than a high school diploma. She did not have a complete idea of what the profession entailed.

Undeterred, Betsy was making inquiries about what qualifications she would need. She talked with chiropractors. She applied to various technical and general colleges to fulfill her undergraduate studies.

One admissions officer with whom she interviewed gave a typical response: "You can't go from being a waitress to a doctor!"

Other interviewers were just as arrogant or discouraging, suggesting that Betsy might settle for a less-professional career. But if you know Betsy, you know she is determined and won't take "no" for an answer.

"I realized that the only way to achieve my dream of becoming a doctor was to move back home with my parents for two years and do my undergraduate work at a local college," says Betsy.

She was accepted into the college and made up the math and science courses that she had missed in high school.

It was going to be a big challenge. Not only did she not have some of the necessary education, but she also would be competing with people ten years younger than she, people who were in the studying habit. Moreover, she had to move away from home and leave her son with her parents back on the farm during the week.

At first, her parents thought the idea was just another of Betsy's ideas—another in the long line of milestones in Betsy's search for a purpose in her life. But they agreed to the plan that would make them surrogate parents of a teenage son, five days a week.

Betsy had doubts, but no doubt that she would succeed. She hadn't studied for years, and she still had to take the science courses she had not even thought about in high school.

She started making up for her lost time by getting friends to teach her algebra, math, and physics. And Betsy had the right attitude. If she didn't know something, she was never afraid to ask. Betsy was also downright competitive and simply wasn't going to allow herself to be left behind. She wasn't. She studied as long as it took, not just to keep up but also to stay at the head of her class. It might take her five hours to do what would only take her younger colleagues one hour, but she was determined.

After two years of undergraduate study, Betsy returned to the Twin Cities to attend a three-and-a-half-year program at the Chiropractic University. This still meant commuting home on weekends to see her son who was living with his grandparents. Betsy's parents never had any doubts that Betsy would succeed once they saw the difference in their daughter and recognized her incredible determination.

Once she had settled into her college courses, Betsy began to enjoy the partying and the activity of daily college life—during the week. During weekends she went home to study and be a mom again.

So this is how Betsy transformed herself from a waitress to a doctor. But there was a price to pay and, ironically, given her former profession, it had to do with food.

When Betsy was in her third year at college, a professor approached her. He wondered whether Betsy had thought about losing some weight. After all, doctors were meant to be role models. Indeed Betsy had been learning all about healthy nutrition, the benefits of exercise, the necessity of a balanced lifestyle, and the risks of obesity. Unfortunately, she wasn't practicing what she was trained to preach. She was nearly forty pounds overweight, and she hadn't noticed.

The professor was an icon in his profession as well as Betsy's mentor. "I was elated that he even noticed me. I knew that I had a problem," says Betsy.

The professor suggested a program supplemented with appetite suppressants, but Betsy was probably doing the program more to impress her professor than to make changes for herself. So while she tried, Betsy was still in denial and made no real changes in her behavior or, consequently, her weight.

Betsy continued, overweight and somewhat embarrassed but simply too focused on her studies and her son to do anything about it. At one time she saw herself on video demonstrating chiropractic technique and although it created some shame and embarrassment, neither were enough to motivate her into action. She had to study, after all.

Betsy graduated after completing her externship. She was soon married and not long after that started to design her own wellness clinic. By now, she was nearly seventy pounds overweight.

The reality of her weight problem finally struck in an undramatic setting. Betsy was shopping with an overweight niece. They were sharing a dressing room, trying on some pants, when it finally hit her! She was wearing the same size as her niece—a size twenty-two.

For someone whose teens were marked by constant concern about the reactions of her community, her next thought was none too surprising: "What will people think?" is the reaction she recalls. Then, "I need to be an example," she thought.

Betsy was now motivated, and there was no turning back. But would she really get going?

"I was definitely resisting, even then," Betsy recalls. "I would spend my time making the house perfect. Then I would be taking care of my husband. Then I had Chad's graduation to consider."

In retrospect Betsy realizes what happened to her: "I was also afraid I wouldn't be able to do it."

Betsy, afraid of failure? Despite all she had achieved, she realized that her weight was going to be her biggest challenge. Her success had always come from single-minded application. Would she be able to apply that to herself without feeling guilty?

"I was feeling guilty about putting me first. As women we almost never put ourselves first," she says. "It's not how we are raised."

Betsy generally achieves her goals regardless of the obstacles—or maybe even because of them. *The day after her son graduated from high school*, Betsy started on her program—the program of putting herself first.

She started to exercise. She eliminated fat from her diet. She stopped people from sabotaging her. "I wasn't afraid to say, 'I can't eat that,'" she says.

T e r r i f i c   T a c t i c

Betsy actively stopped people from getting her off her program by forthrightly saying that she couldn't eat various foods no matter who gave them to her and what the context.

And she didn't feel guilty.

She started a weight-loss group in her wellness center, and twelve people joined that night. Within nine months, she had lost sixty-six pounds.

"It was hard, but finding out who I really was made the effort worthwhile. The rewards I got for being healthy far outweighed the sacrifices I had to make. I had to give up being an athlete in school when I got pregnant at fifteen, but now I have that part of me back again. Not having to struggle consciously and unconsciously with the heavy burden of weight is tremendously liberating," she says.

Today, Betsy is vibrant and happy. You feel that at last she has her life in balance.

"Because I was able to put myself first and find happiness within myself, I am now a better mom, wife, and friend," she says.

Now she takes satisfaction and meaning in giving back to her clients and her group members. Their pain is a reminder of her own experiences and keeps her in touch with her own experience and motivation.

"I'm here for my life, and that's okay," says Betsy, echoing a major theme of her motivational seminars.

Life isn't about finding yourself, life is about creating yourself. – George Bernard Shaw

A Promise Fulfilled—Barbara Konwinski

*Barbara Konwinski has had her share of adversity. This turned
her into a fatalist, who used food to cope, with a hearty denial of
what her eating was doing to her. These are her words.*

I have always had a weight problem. I come from a heavy family. Both parents and my three siblings were all overweight. I was teased at school, but I tried not to let it bother me. I have an outgoing personality, so I tried not to let the sarcastic comments and social exclusion get the better of me. It was especially awkward when adolescence hit. I had friends but still did not feel normal or on a par with my classmates. I felt like a failure.

During my college years, I had small success on a number of diets, but the weight would always come back. I was a sneak eater, often bingeing in private and feeling very ashamed and guilty about it. Not long after graduating college, I fulfilled my childhood dream and became an elementary school teacher. Spurred on by the thought of my responsibility, I started to exercise but was still eating heavily. When three years later I met the man of my dreams, I was really inspired to do something about my eating and lost forty pounds prior to our marriage.

Over the next twenty years, my weight crept back on. There were the usual ups and downs, and I gave birth to two boys. During this time I became concerned about my weight, but never concerned enough to want to do anything about it. And then a series of events happened that made me feel as if there was nothing I *could* do about it.

First, my husband lost his job when his company relocated. This was a considerable financial blow and really disrupted us. Our two boys were just becoming teenagers and did not need this dislocation. My husband was stressed out, and that made life difficult all 'round.

Then, on Christmas day, our van caught fire. It was in the driveway and before we could control it, the fire spread to the house. We managed to evacuate the two boys and the dog, but when it was all over, half our house was gone. All three television stations came to cover that local tragedy. We had to live with my mother for four months while our house was repaired.

Finally, my eldest son, who had always been a free spirit and given us a lot of challenges, was paralyzed in an automobile accident. Needless to say, seeing your firstborn confined to a wheelchair for the rest of his life as a quadriplegic is devastating beyond description.

After each setback I turned to food for temporary comfort and relief. I didn't care that I was adding to my already-burdened frame. I didn't feel there was much I could do about that anyway. Actually, I was feeling that I couldn't do much about anything. I was out of control and completely fatalistic.

By 1997, my weight had ballooned to an all-time high of 268 pounds. I could barely walk from the parking lot to the store without getting breathless. Deep down I knew something was wrong, but I kept telling myself that I was just "out of shape." I must have been worried enough because I joined TOPS and started going to meetings. I still had my doubts that I could lose the weight and give up my eating habits. By this time, I was on medication for high blood pressure and diabetes.

After I had been going to TOPS for a few weeks, I had lost a little weight but was still feeling out of breath. I went back to my doctor and after several tests he told me the news: I needed quintuple bypass surgery. I was forty-seven years old.

My mother had required a quadruple bypass a year earlier. She had a heart attack, waited six hours before calling anyone, and her heart was damaged. Fatalism must be genetic.

My father had died of heart disease at the age of fifty-five, several years earlier. On his deathbed he had taken my hand, looked straight into my eyes, and made me promise to do something about my weight. Of course, I hadn't. I hadn't because I didn't think I could. But now I was having to rethink.

As I lay recovering from my successful bypass surgery, it finally struck me. Through the years, I had somehow allowed all the events that had happened to me to control me. I became paralyzed by them as much as my son was paralyzed by his automobile accident. Bad things happened, I ate, gained weight, and retreated into my corner, defeated and helpless. Oh sure, I did not fold completely, was functional, and managed to survive. But I had turned into a victim—passive and unwilling or incapable of taking charge.

Now things were different, however. Through prayer and the support and encouragement of family, friends, students, and TOPS pals, I decided I had to find a way to take control of my physical behavior and my emotions. It was do that or die.

The first thing I did was to make exercise a part of my everyday life. I started by walking 'round and 'round my dining table. How ironic that I turned a dining table into an exercise track! Once I got stronger, I started walking up and down my driveway. Before long I progressed to the mall. Now I walk three miles every day with my mom and alternate Tae-Bo, resistance exercises, line dancing, water aerobics, and biking every evening. I never believed that I would ever enjoy exercise, but I do. And I try to persuade others to join me.

Terrific   Tactic

Think "movement," not exercise. Barbara started out by simply moving more around her house and was able to graduate to more-structured exercise.

I also took charge of my eating habits. I wrote down everything I ate, drank eight glasses of water a day, and started eating three meals a day. I never used to eat breakfast and would graze throughout the day, but I don't do that anymore.

T e r r i f i c   T a c t i c

Eat breakfast. If you don't, you run the risk that your blood-glucose level will sink very low and set off strong hunger or even cravings later in the day.

In 1998 I lost eighty-eight pounds. I now have lost a total of 120 pounds and am down to a size ten. I am no longer on medication for high blood pressure or diabetes. I have never felt better, either physically or emotionally.

When I first walked into that TOPS group in the fall of 1997, I was embarrassed and ashamed. For the first year I wore the same clothes to every meeting. But the support and care I got from TOPS was overwhelming. But perhaps what I got most of all was empowerment. What I got was the positive attitude and the idea that I did control my own destiny.

Now I can talk to the parents of my third-grade students who show the signs of chubbiness and awkwardness that I experienced. I have found that parents and children alike welcome my comments and can learn from my experiences.

I can hold my head up now, and sometimes I look skyward and see my dad looking down. Finally, I have kept my promise to him.

No price is too high to pay for the privilege
of owning yourself. – Friedrich Wilhelm Nietsche

Paying Attention—Roe WiersGalla

Roe WiersGalla spent much of her adult life oscillating between pre-contemplation and the next stage, contemplation. For Roe, pre-contemplation initially manifested itself as indifference but later turned into helplessness. This is her story.

I can't really explain why I was overweight as a child. Neither my parents nor any of my four brothers were overweight. My mother was one of fifteen, none of whom had weight problems, and my father also had no family history of obesity. I had a great childhood. I never really thought of myself as fat when a child, and if I did get teased, I don't recall being affected by it. My father mentioned my weight to me once, but apart from that, no one in the family addressed the issue with me at all. This, despite the fact that by the time I reached early adulthood I was a little over five feet tall and weighed over two hundred pounds.

After school, I took a job as an office manager for a law firm and have been doing that with one firm or another for the past thirty-five years. In my early adult life, I was somewhat concerned about my weight. Over about ten years, I tried a dozen different diets. I did lose sixty pounds by fasting once, but then I relocated and couldn't find anyone to administer my program. As on every other occasion, I quickly put the weight back on. I found backsliding easy. One time I was into an exercise program. My exercise cycle broke, and that was the end of that!

By the time I reached my early thirties, I stopped worrying about my weight. It did not seem to be affecting my life at all. I had a good social life, my career was blossoming, and my health was good. I stopped paying it any attention.

For the next ten years, I continued flourishing, socially and occupationally. While I hadn't been paying attention, my weight had climbed to over three hundred pounds. Then, in my mid-forties, I did start to get some discomfort from it. I was getting irritated by having to get my business suits custom made. Certain car seats were uncomfortable, and I began to sense the limitations of my weight. But now as I thought about my weight I was terrified. I didn't think I could lose it. Somehow, over the years, my indifference had turned into helplessness.

So I stopped thinking about it.

Another few years passed before I started thinking about it again. My legs started to swell. The discoloration and mottled appearance of my calf, which I saw every day, did not even scare me. It was only four years later that I began to take notice.

I had developed a small skin ulcer on my leg. At first, I thought it was nothing. But when it didn't go away after six weeks, I started to get really worried. My mother had died of cancer of the liver, and I thought the fact that my ulcer was not healing was a sign that I had cancer. Finally, I made an appointment to see the doctor.

I could tell you that my reticence to go to a physician was due to the fact that for many years I had worked for a legal firm that specialized in medical malpractice. My confidence in physicians was not very high! Looking back, I can see that this was an excuse. The plain fact of the matter is that I was terrified. I weighed 365 pounds and had already decided that I was going to die at this weight.

I changed the medical appointment twice. I eventually summoned up the courage to actually keep the appointment at St. Luke's Hospital in Milwaukee, which I knew to be one of the best. I couldn't have gotten a better doctor. Dr. Milka Mandich diagnosed me as having Peripheral Vascular Disease. She ran a variety of tests. My cholesterol was over 270. Other test results came back remarkably and surprisingly normal. I needed treatment, however. If I didn't get it, I would run the real risk of losing my leg.

The treatment was, of course, to lose weight. Dr. Mandich did not threaten, cajole, or coerce me. She must have known that would not have worked on me, even in my precarious medical condition. Instead, she gave me hope, support, and a plan. She sent me to the nutritionist and gave me an exercise plan that started with five minutes a day in my chair.

Within two months I had lost thirty pounds, and my cholesterol was down to 180. But the real challenge was how to keep this going. How was I going to maintain my effort?

Looking back now, I find it funny how I missed the signs that were in front of me all the time. For four years, I looked at my discolored legs every day and had chosen not to see what that meant. And every day for twenty years I had been passing TOPS national headquarters in Milwaukee and not even considered exploring their possibilities. But now it was time and, summoning up my courage yet again, I ventured into my first TOPS meeting.

I knew immediately that the support, inspiration, and information I found there would be a great help. I followed a broad but balanced food plan, lowered my fat intake, and drank at least a dozen glasses of water daily. I did not and still do not miss my weekly TOPS meeting or my monthly visit to the nutritionist. The accountability of going to the meetings and my journal were critical in getting me on track.

Terrific Tactic

Accountability, accountability, accountability. Roe used not only her group but also a regular visit to a health professional—in her case, a nutritionist—to ensure that she stayed on track.

My exercise increased from those few minutes a day from my chair.

In the first few months I was using low-impact aerobic tapes. When, after eight months, I had lost more than ninety pounds, my osteoarthritis in my knee improved, and I was able to walk outside and to lift weights.

In the first few months I was getting my clothes altered almost weekly. Within a year, I threw them all out and bought myself a new wardrobe. By then I didn't need a size fifty-four. Today I wear a size fourteen.

Two years after I started out on what I then considered an impossible journey, I reached my goal. My physician had prescribed a goal of two hundred pounds, but I felt more comfortable getting down to 190—an overall loss of 175 pounds.

In the beginning, I was secretive about my weight-control efforts. It wasn't until I had lost about a hundred pounds that people started to notice the change. People who hadn't seen me for a while did not recognize me. I didn't recognize me. I didn't believe I would ever walk without pain. I didn't ever believe that I would actually want to exercise. I didn't ever believe I could lose the weight.

I regret that I didn't make the choice to lose the weight ten years sooner. I wasn't ready to believe that I could do it. In the end, with the help of my doctor, nutritionist, and TOPS friends, I was able to make the choice and take control of my life. Better late than never!

An Overall Change—Chuck Barber

*Chuck Barber describes a classic case of resistance and denial.
His defense was initially penetrated by the fact that the only
coworker of similar size—a man who had lent Chuck overalls—
dropped dead of a heart attack almost in front of Chuck's very
eyes. Even then, Chuck's resistance continued, until he eventually
found the courage and support to make a positive choice.*

I have been big most of my life — big in all the wrong places. Growing up in the 1950s and 60s there weren't near as many overweight children, so quite often I found myself being the only "fat kid" on the block or in my class at school. President Kennedy's physical fitness program for children, in the early 60s, was just one more opportunity for me to fail. I was just too heavy to do pushups or pull ups, and run a mile. Who are you kidding? Sometimes I would stand in the bathroom in front of the mirror and wonder why I was the one chosen to be so big. Because of my size I was the target of a lot of name calling and beatings; usually several boys from school would follow me home calling me "fatso" and other names; then when I would turn to confront them, they would beat me. One particularly painful memory from elementary school days revolves around Valentine's Day. It seems the teacher wanted to pair us off for dancing, the only problem being that none of the girls wanted to be the partner of the "fat guy."

During my adolescence, I was really involved in sports, sometimes to the point of excluding time for trying to have relationships with girls. Sports became my escape hatch and motivator. My coaches ran me to death trying to get the weight off of me, with a great deal of success. However, when I got hurt or the season was over, the motivation was gone. I was usually pretty shy around the girls at all times because most of them could only see me as the fat guy, and I couldn't seem to get beyond that self-image. When a girl would express an interest in me, I would withdraw from her until she lost interest because I was so afraid of possible rejection.

During my sophomore year in high school, I broke my left leg playing football. Complications of the fracture left me in a body cast and subsequently with osteoarthritis. Since I was basically an active person, the combination of excess weight, arthritis, and activity started to cause a lot of pain and stiffness, eventually leading to my discharge from the Navy as a 10 percent disabled veteran. I began to notice that during cold and damp periods some of my joints would swell until they were almost useless. Also I began to experience severe back problems. One particular time my back was so bad that I had to roll out of bed and crawl to the phone to call my wife. Several doctors, orthopedic surgeons, and rheumatologists told me weight loss was the only real remedy to this problem.

By the time I was twenty, married, and in the Navy I was already an experienced yo-yo dieter, having lost and regained significant weight three times. By this time I was so big that most of the guys didn't really try to bully me, and I was so into trying to fit in that I entered into the joking about my size. As a DJ on the AFRTS radio station aboard ship, my handle became "Mongo," the big dumb guy from *Blazing Saddles*. Mostly the guys wanted to challenge me to see if they could take on a guy who outweighed them by one hundred pounds or more. I spent six years in the Navy at a variety of duty stations including two tours in Vietnam aboard the USS Constellation. During this time I got larger and larger; at one point, during my time in Hospital Corps school, my classmates discovered that adipose tissue was another way to say fat, so that became my nickname. Within a few years of my medical discharge I weighed an uncomfortable 360 pounds, and I needed help. It got so bad that my daughter and I were turned away from a roller coaster ride at the amusement park because I was simply too big; of course, everyone in line laughed at me as we departed.

My daughter also had to endure the pain of having her friends laugh at me and call me names in front of her. I remember that my son once had an assignment in school for Father's Day, to write and illustrate a story along the lines of "What my Dad is to me." His story and illustration showed me sitting in my chair, watching TV, with a bag of chips. Yes, I was a couch potato; I was too ashamed of myself to go out in public if I could get away from it. I didn't even go to many of my children's school events.

As I grew older, I noticed that there were more and more obese people, some even on TV—e.g., John Madden—so I started to rationalize by comparing myself to others. I would look at another fat person and say, "At least I am not that big." There were clothing stores for big and tall people, and I figured as long as I wasn't wearing the largest sizes they had I must be OK.

I became a yo-yo dieter, and my wife may have suffered the most of all. She never knew what to expect from me. During my all-too-brief skinny periods, I was energetic and willing to go places with her. However, when my weight was back up, I would withdraw and become depressed. Going out to dinner meant takeout and eating in front of the TV. My emotions were also on a roller coaster, and I would often get very angry for no real reason.

When I was overweight, I was an extremely negative and sometimes depressed person. Some of my friends at work said that I was a "glass is half empty" kind of person. I wore my feelings on my sleeve, and almost any small upset could send me into a rage or a fit of depression.

Over the next several years, I lied to myself about the weight gain, ever-expanding waistline, and decreasing mobility due to all that weight on arthritic joints. When I went for a driver's license, I told them I weighed 250 pounds and was shocked at my doctor's office a month later to see the scale read 280. So I did what I had always done when depressed about my weight: I ate more.

When I started a new job in 1995, I had to borrow overalls until mine arrived; I was so big that only one man in the whole shop had any to fit me. By the summer of 1998, I was back up to 320 pounds and really starting to feel it. About this time the same man who loaned me his overalls got sick at work one night—he complained of back pain, so we all thought he had hurt his back. I helped him into a van for him to drive home. The next morning, his wife discovered he had passed away of a heart attack in bed. We were all shocked, and I started thinking that I really did not want my wife to find me dead of a heart attack in our bed. At least not this young. I had a choice to make.

Having lost and regained weight so many times, I really did not want to get involved in another weight-loss program, which I felt sure would fail. However, the choice was either become an invalid or do something about it. The realization that, at forty-eight, I should be able to do a lot more than I was, and fear of being confined to a desk job or maybe even a wheelchair if I did not do something, gave me the courage I needed to overcome my apathy.

I contacted TOPS and received a letter telling me where and when the meetings were. That thing made a great bookmark and place to put my coffee cup down, but apparently it won't help you lose weight unless you actually attend the meetings. So, I finally stopped putting it off and got enough courage to attend a meeting in San Jose. I really had no idea what to expect, although I imagined it would be much of the same empty rhetoric and financially taxing hype I had encountered at so many other places. I was still resistant and reluctant.

As I sat there, I was feeling really out of place, especially when they paraded all the members of the group who had successfully lost weight and maintained the loss. I had doubts that I could ever get this weight off again because I had never maintained a loss, but there was no gracious way out.

I was also the only man in the room, and that was only one of the challenges. I discovered that TOPS had no specific program for me to follow. I was going to have to actually give it some thought. No one was going to spoon feed me information and provide me with menus or prepared meals. I did discover that TOPS people are committed to one another; they support and assist each other not only in weight loss but also in all the areas of life that contribute to stress and emotional eating.

I was made to feel not only welcome but also included in the group, and that made a huge difference and began to turn my attitude around. During our roll calls, when each member announces her weight loss or gain for the week, the leader would ask me how I accomplished my loss for the week, and as I shared I could feel my self-confidence rising. Every week when I got off the scale, the other members were just as enthused about my success as I was. Those in my chapter have cheered for all of my successes and helped me to face any setbacks in a calm and rational manner. I learned that I have value as a part of the group for who I am, not just what I look like. *This level of support is exactly what I needed to come out of my shell.*

My family and friends were real helpful. Patty made sure that we always had the right foods in the house, and my friends were willing to put up with having to provide me with alternate foods at cookouts and get-togethers so I could participate and not feel left out.

Terrific Tactic

Chuck ensured that there were healthy foods available at social gatherings so that he could participate socially and not feel tempted or isolated.

Seeing the scale move downward, and being rewarded for that progress, really kept me going. Starting at 320 pounds, I made steady progress until I reached my goal of 225 pounds. Thanks to the Exchange diet, exercise, and drinking at least a hundred ounces of water daily, I have lost ninety-four pounds and kept it off.

Since losing weight, I have felt a stability that was never there before. I no longer let events and people control my emotions. It is much easier now to look at a situation and determine a reasonable course of action as opposed to just reacting negatively to it.

I now have the tools needed to succeed at this new lifestyle. First, and most important, I have learned that this is not a diet but a change in my lifestyle and my way of thinking. I also realize the incredible value of support and successful role models in giving hope.

I have developed a couple of strategies to help me maintain my loss. After my weigh-in each week I do two things: I set a goal to be at or below goal the next week, and I visualize my plan to achieve that goal. I see myself succeeding.

Terrific Tactic

Chuck sets weekly weight goals. Short-term goals are good in that they can provide a daily incentive.

I have made the choice to succeed.

My Eyes Have Been Opened
—Inez Ferrara

Inez Ferrara describes how severe sight impairment drove her into helplessness until she found the strength from within and from others to stage a remarkable recovery.

My mother had the same condition. She lived to be ninety-three, but the last twenty years of her life were a complete misery. She lived in almost complete isolation, frozen in a bleak tundra of self-pity. I hated what it did to her and how she reacted. I was never going to be like that. Anyway, I wasn't even going to get the condition.

I was wrong on both counts.

By the time I was officially diagnosed as being legally blind with macular degeneration, I was completely blind in my left eye and could only make out some shapes and shadows in my right. Even though it had been coming for some time, I couldn't see it. Blind emotionally and literally. When that realization finally arrived, however, it was a huge emotional shock. I was numb. I have always been an active, independent person, and now I came face to face with my limitations. I was very dependent on my friends and family. My husband was extraordinarily supportive and protective, but I'd much rather he not be in that position. Gone was the traveling which was so much a part of my life.

So I started knitting, getting lots of audio books, and eating sweets. Lots of sweets. To say that I felt sorry for myself is an understatement. Why me? Why now? Not fair! Don't care! I was immobilized by my self-pity. My weight, which was already high, inched up as my spirits went down.

I was having difficulty controlling my weight and my mood despite the efforts of my friends and TOPS pals, but I just didn't care. After all, I couldn't see myself, and when you lose your sight, appearance doesn't much matter any more. I didn't have to avoid mirrors and videos of myself. Nature had taken care of that for me.

My turning point came when I attended a TOPS State Recognition Day. As my friends made their way down the aisles, showing off their handiwork, my blindness really hit me. Here I was, sitting amid all the excitement and fun, and I could see nothing. I felt helpless and isolated. I was so overcome that I rushed to the restroom and locked myself in a stall, sobbing. It was there that I realized that I could not go on like this any longer. It was time to take control of my life again.

Prompted by this epiphany and the encouragement of my friends, I decided to visit the Lighthouse for the Blind, a facility that helped the unsighted with independent living skills. Going to such a place meant no longer denying the extent of my condition. I was a little apprehensive about my visit.

What I saw there shocked me. Yes, I was still able to see some. What I saw and heard were people far worse off than me. Many people had no vision at all. Others had no vision and no support either. Others had no vision, no support, and other crippling conditions, too. None of them were complaining. None of them were feeling sorry for themselves. All of them were doing the best they could under their given circumstances. I felt ashamed, embarrassed, and inspired. The Lighthouse was a beacon, and it was showing me the way home.

I went to the Lighthouse for four-and-a-half months. I learned how to work the special software that made it possible to use a computer. I started typing and cooking. I also started doing something about my weight.

I eliminated fried food from my diet completely, so much so that I no longer have a taste for it at all. I stopped the ice cream desserts and snacks and switched to frozen yogurt. I got a talking scale to measure portions. I have difficulty in keeping track of calories because I can't easily write down what I have eaten, but I still manage by memorizing my food intake and simply being aware of it.

Inez eliminated fried food completely. Total abstinence is easier than perfect moderation. Fried food is not a nutritional necessity. Eliminate it.

I had now grabbed life by the throat. I volunteered at the Youth Center for a while, and now I volunteer at Tampa General Hospital. I continue to cook, type, and be active in the community. And I've lost about fifty pounds.

Being visually challenged has taught me several valuable lessons. I've learned the value of patience. I've learned that there is more to life than appearance. Most of all, I've learned to be grateful for what I have. I've resumed traveling. Museums are a waste of time for me, but landscapes aren't. You could say that I have got the big picture.

Do what you can, with what you have, where you are . – Theodore Roosevelt

Rankin's Reminders

Power Generators

Manage time. Don't commit your time without thinking about whether this is draining or enhancing.

Know your friends. Make a list of those who empower you and those who disempower you. Avoid the latter, if possible.

Be assertive. Don't be afraid to say no!

Determine what situations make you feel helpless. How can you cope with these better, i.e., other than eating?

Be proactive. Recognize that difficulty is not the same as helplessness.

Define your boundaries. Know limits of where and how far others can encroach.

Don't sulk or whine. Self-pity, doubt, and fear will erode your choices.

Notes

---

[1] Information about the Exchange System can be obtained by calling TOPS at 1-800-932-8677.

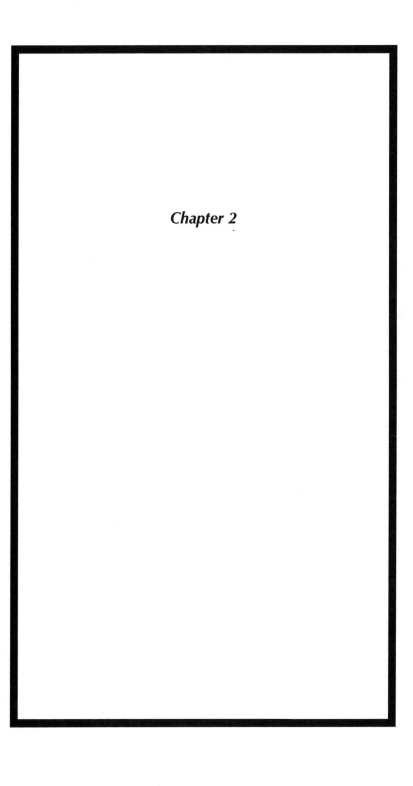

Chapter 2

Changing Vision

Improve self-esteem

It's hard to fight an enemy who has outposts
in your head. – Sally Kempton

A burdened soul leads to a burdened body.

Carrying excess weight can severely damage your self-esteem, but the reverse is equally true. Low self-image is a precursor to weight gain and obesity. That does not mean that every woman with poor self-image is overweight or that you have to have low self-esteem to be overweight. There are several examples in this book of women who were significantly overweight but appeared to have a healthy level of self-regard. Low self-esteem is so pervasive in its destructive effects, however, that it severely restricts the ability to successfully manage a weight problem.

The basis of self-image is formed in childhood. Children do not have the mental abilities to rationally evaluate what is said to them, and because it is imperative that they view their parents as all knowing and all powerful, anything that is said to a child—especially a young child—*has to be believed* as true. Children thus walk around in something akin to a hypnotic state, uncritically absorbing messages, spoken and nonspoken, from all adults—but especially from parents.

Moreover, most children will assume responsibility for their parents. Parents are the child's lifeline; therefore, it is critical that they are kept stable and well. This responsibility is the default setting for most children. If dad is an alcoholic, then it becomes the child's responsibility to prevent drinking; if mom is depressed, then it becomes the child's responsibility to keep her happy. This mistaken association between the child's behavior and the parent's actions can create not only the burden of responsibility in the child but also an overwhelming sense of failure. Children don't know it, but their behavior has very little effect on their parents. Naively, they are trying to control the uncontrollable. As a result, it is not just abuse and negativity that create self-esteem problems. Immature, moody, and uncontrolled behavior from parents has the same effect.

Once the "master tapes" of self-doubt, lack of confidence, and self-deprecation are dubbed into the mind, they influence all perceptions. The world is seen through the lens of low self-worth, which distorts even the most positive comments. For example, people with low self-esteem frequently cannot accept compliments. Because the compliment is inconsistent with the poor view of themselves, it has to be rejected. Such people will squirm uncomfortably when they get a compliment, trying to reject it out of hand or rationalizing it away as insincere.

When our behavior is inconsistent with our beliefs and attitudes, we feel very uncomfortable. Our experience is filtered through our self-esteem and is created to be consistent with it. The toxic influence of low self-esteem can thus spread to all corners of the mind. If you think negatively of yourself, all other experience has to be consistent with that view. It's not possible to feel negatively about your spirit while feeling positively about your appearance.

Poor self-image spreads its malign effect beyond just appearance, however, and projects onto all other personal characteristics. Poor eating and health habits are consistent with poor self-image; to maintain poor self-image *they have to be.* Poor body image and poor health habits are not just a consequence of low self-esteem, *they are also a requirement for it.*

If you want further demonstration that self-esteem can distort body image, you need look no further than the local eating disorders unit. There you will find anorexics who genuinely believe that their emaciated bodies are fat. They have to believe that their bodies are fat because most anorexics are failing perfectionists who are constantly struggling with control. Their self-image requires them to be battling for control, something that would not be necessary if they did not see themselves as fat. Hence, they have to retain an image of being fat even when they are emaciated. There are few more puzzling and frustrating clinical experiences than seeing an anorexic judge her fatally thin body as fat, and yet happily and realistically agree that the girl standing next to them weighing forty pounds more is "just right." In this book, you will read of people who still literally see themselves as fat even when the scales and everyone else around them tell them otherwise.

Low self-esteem is often defined by feelings of emptiness, loneliness, and complete frustration. Because low self-esteem precludes positive, or even any, social interaction—the very thing that helps self-esteem the most—positive contact with other people is not available. That leaves few alternatives to assuage chronic painful feelings. Those that are left are simple physical remedies that temporarily cover up the discomfort—alcohol, drugs, and food.

So both poor eating and the consequent weight gain are a confirmation of low self-esteem.

The way you talk to yourself is the way you talk to others. People with low self-esteem are constantly criticizing themselves. This poor self-perception obviously influences others who then reinforce this negative view. A classic example of the axiom that you only get treated the way you ask to be treated.

Poor self-esteem does not just impact thoughts; it significantly affects mood and behavior, too. Negativity is heavy; it is tiring to carry it around. It is burdensome and affects posture. It creates mental and physical fatigue. I believe that biology is a reflection of biography and that heaviness of spirit goes hand in hand with heaviness of body. In many of the stories in this book, people report feeling unburdened by losing their weight. They feel lighter not just because they have lost their physical weight, but also because they have shed their spiritual burdens.

Self-defeating thoughts lead to social isolation. Social interaction can be a painful, constant reminder of inadequacy and failure. Hardly surprising, therefore, that many choose to hide. Some do this by becoming socially phobic and isolated. Others cannot easily escape, and so they build their own camouflage, choosing to remain hidden under a canopy of fat cells. Excess weight is a barrier to social interaction—a Berlin wall designed to keep others out. When others are kept out, you are shut in.

The symptoms of low self-esteem conspire to prevent any successful weight loss.

- First, being overweight and having poor health habits is consistent with a poor self-image.

- Second, food and alcohol, both weight enhancers, provide easy, if only temporary, relief from the feelings of inadequacy.

- Third, negativity and lack of confidence doom any project as demanding as lifestyle change.

- Fourth, those with low self-esteem simply don't have the mental and physical energy to devote to changing their eating habits and embarking on a worthwhile exercise program.

- Fifth, losing weight means giving up the camouflage under which many with poor self-worth hide. It is hardly surprising that so many fail so often.

In the geography of emotions, low self-esteem shares a border with self-pity. It is easy to stray across this border and feel badly *for* yourself because you feel badly *about* yourself. Self-pity is the enemy of action. Venture into the vast hinterland of self-pity and you risk being lost forever in the jungles of bitterness and the swamps of misdirected sorrow.

So, how can one escape the self-fulfilling bind of low self-esteem?

Low self-esteem is born out of negative social interaction and can only be restored through positive interaction. Who are the right people that can help restore self-esteem, and what do you need from them?

One individual can make a huge difference, especially when he occupies a major role in your life. It almost always takes several people, however, working either individually or as a team, to begin the long process of restoring confidence and elevating self-worth. The key elements of this recovery process are as follows.

- The prime requirement of an esteem restorer is to show unconditional acceptance. The person with low self-esteem needs no invitation to play a critical tune. A healing individual or group will provide no such opportunity. On the contrary, the right group of people will not only *not* judge this person, but it also will have a totally nonjudgmental philosophy and aura. This is essential and quite unnatural. Almost all relationships are conditional and judgmental, which traps the unconfident and those who assume failure. An atmosphere of unconditional acceptance is an absolute requisite for changing low self-esteem.

- In addition, the effective group provides successful role models that can inspire hope and optimism. A group that contains members who have experienced low self-esteem and who have overcome such problems will be especially powerful.

- The group also needs to credibly challenge toxic and self-defeating thoughts and behaviors. This is by far the most significant type of support that anyone can give. Most of us are prone to losing our perspective when things go wrong. What prevents us from going off track is feedback that restores a more adaptive, realistic, and optimistic viewpoint. In my experience, the biggest factor differentiating successes from failures in weight-management programs is the ability of the successes to get back on track after being derailed. The failures almost uniformly see the first slip as evidence of their inevitable failure and give up.

- An effective group also exposes a dangerous confusion that lies at the heart of all self-esteem problems. It needs to communicate that failure does not make a bad person any more than success makes a good person. Achievement and morality are not to be confused. Unfortunately, we use the same words, "good" and "bad," to measure behavioral success and moral worth. This is the problem of "good"—that it creates horrible confusion, especially in the minds of children, who do not understand the subtleties of semantics. Many enlightened parents today go out of their way to make the distinction between a child's behavior and their moral worth. "It's not that I don't love you; it's that I don't like what you did," is the core of that valuable message. All too frequently adults forget to apply that fundamental principle to their own behavior.

The self-esteem restorers need to do all the above without taking away the person's responsibility for her actions. They encourage the person to try new things, take on positive challenges, and enable her to do what is necessary to reach her goals, *but they never do it for her.*

"Guardian angels" cannot be found on any street corner. Any one person might be able to fulfill all the requirements, but a group is far more powerful than any individual. I believe this is a function that TOPS fulfills extremely well. In virtually every story in this book—and in the dozens of stories I have read that are not included in this book—the unconditional acceptance, lack of judgment, and positive approach of the TOPS members who could identify with the presenting problems was as overwhelming as it was empowering. It is this, say TOPS members, that makes the organization unique and inspires its members' loyalty.

Darkness Fading—Robin Nolan

*Robin Nolan describes how she became completely isolated and
actually socially phobic. When both physical and emotional pain
forced her to reach out, she struggled to find a positive social
connection until she received a hug from a stranger one morning
in an unknown church.*

---

*Robin Nolan was not overweight as a child, despite having parents who were
less than the ideal weight. After enduring a difficult—and at times abusive
and traumatic—childhood, she left the Midwest for California. There she
started a relationship with an older man which was less than satisfying. That's
when the weight started to creep on.*

Robin noticed the weight gain right away but chose to ignore it. She
stopped looking in the mirror. In her mind, she stopped registering her
clothes size. She stopped paying attention, period.

Before long, Robin was in the midst of a full-blown addiction. On
bad days, she would go from one drive-through to another, eventually
accumulating enough food for four people. She would then hurriedly
cover the food with her jacket so no one could see—especially her.

"I felt horrible when I ordered the food and horrible after I'd eaten
it," says Robin.

As food became her drug of choice, Robin would spend more and
more time secluded in her home. Ashamed when she was eating,
ashamed when she wasn't. Trapped in a cycle of despair, seclusion, and
guilt.

"I thought of food from morning until I went to bed in the evening.
My life revolved around food."

Occasionally the pain was so great that Robin would be motivated
to try to break the pattern. But feeling motivated and taking action are

two different stages.

"I would vow each morning that today was the day I wasn't going to binge, but I would start again within a few hours."

For nearly fifteen years, Robin lived this existence. It was suicide by silverware, and she knew it. What was worse, Robin cut herself off from her family. She was now almost completely isolated. Alone in the world with just quarter pounders and fries to keep her company.

She cursorily tried a number of organizations along the way but always dropped out very quickly. In retrospect, that was partly due to her mental state and partly due to the impersonal nature of the programs.

"I was looking for a connection and never really found it," says Robin of her wilderness years. Her relationship was not providing much of a connection either. After fifteen years of ambivalence and indifference, she ended it.

Robin never sought professional help at this time, but if she had she probably would have been diagnosed with an eating disorder and agoraphobia. With her self-esteem and waistline going in opposite directions, Robin knew that somehow she had to change her life.

Following the end of her long-term relationship, Robin spent five years analyzing herself, knowing she had to change but never quite taking the action steps. She started being honest with herself and accepting responsibility for her actions. She began to keep a journal and observed the patterns in her behavior.

This self-analysis was important, but her confidence was still virtually nonexistent. She was still completely isolated and, to make matters worse, she was starting to have chest pains. At one level these symptoms alarmed her. She had a family history of heart problems, but as long as the pains were intermittent, Robin could deny their seriousness. Soon, the symptoms became chronic, and denial was getting more and more difficult.

It was not the chest pain per se that broke through Robin's denial. After all, this was a woman who had been humiliated many times in the past. On one occasion, a complete stranger removed a bag of potato chips from her shopping cart with the admonition, "You don't need these." Robin just left the cart and fled. On another occasion, a woman mooed at her mockingly as she entered and then left a local store. People would hold the door open for others but not for her. Social humiliation was one thing; physical limitations were another. She was unable to walk more than twenty feet without feeling exhausted.

So Robin was no stranger to shame and pain. But the chest pains came at a time when she was opening herself up to outside influence. Ending an unsatisfying relationship was the start. Now she was hesitatingly reaching out to the rest of the world. The first place she turned was to a higher power. She started to see the events in her life as signs from God.

"I kept having daily thoughts about finding an organization that would truly make a difference in my life. I came to the conclusion that isolation was too painful. With chest pains daily, I had to face the fact that I could decide to live or die. I decided I wanted to live," says Robin.

So, the chest pains weren't just chest pains.

With ambivalence, fear, and reluctance, Robin searched for the local TOPS chapter number.

"Even when I got the information, I just put it aside and ate," remembers Robin.

A week later she decided to attend the Thursday morning meeting at a group twenty-five miles away in Redding.

"I remember telling myself to turn 'round and go back home because TOPS is not going to make any difference."

After taking a very circuitous route, Robin literally found herself at the meeting place. Fittingly, it was The Community Church of God—another sign perhaps? And she was there at 7:30 A.M. for a 9 A.M. meeting. When Robin finally plucked up enough courage to walk into the meeting, she was welcomed with open arms and a hug.

"That hug meant a lot to me. I had arrived so early because I was ashamed and didn't want to be seen. When I got that hug, I knew I had found a place where I was not going to be judged for my size or my appearance. We were all in the same boat. We all had a need for fellowship and understanding of the ultimate control food had over us," recalls Robin.

She was then directed to the scales. At 300 pounds, the scales did not move. At 350 pounds they did not move either. The weight recorder told Robin that she could not be weighed this week but would be at the next meeting.

With a week of reprieve, Robin took full advantage of not having to start her "diet" for another week. More importantly, she did go back the next week. The warmth and acceptance she had found at the first meeting exceeded her wildest expectations.

The next week the scales were adapted with the addition of a fishing weight, and Robin tipped the scales at 402 pounds.

"I was breathless. I was determined to get rid of that darned fishing weight," says Robin.

It took her eight weeks to get rid of the first fishing weight. It took her four more weeks to get rid of the second one. Everyone cheered when Robin could be weighed without "outside assistance." Everyone cheered when the scale moved from the 350- to the 300-pound level. There was more cheering when she moved down to 250.

Robin is almost apologetic when she explains that if you have to cut back from ten thousand calories a day, as she did, it is not difficult to lose weight. She monitored every portion of her food intake meticulously, drank plenty of water, and started to exercise. And she never missed a weekly meeting. But none of that would not have been possible without the unconditional acceptance Robin received in the group.

T e r r i f i c   T a c t i c

**Robin measured every portion of food meticulously. This is
essential, at least in the beginning. It is the norm to deceive
yourself about the amount of food you are eating.**

"I went in thinking I was going to be judged, but I was wrong," says
Robin.

When others don't judge you, they are showing that judgment is
unnecessary. When others don't judge you, they are teaching you how
to accept yourself. For the first time, Robin was able to ease up on herself. She really had found a family.

"TOPS became my extended family. We share many things and support each other in so many ways. We walk together. We talk together.
We share the joy and the pain of each others' lives," says Robin.

Although Robin was recognized as one of the most successful members after she lost sixty-four pounds, she still did not comprehend the
enormity of her pending transformation.

"It was not until I lost a hundred pounds that I noticed physical
changes. It was not until I lost 150 pounds that I started to look in the
mirror," says Robin.

There were other changes. When she was down 150 pounds, a man
helped her as she struggled with some shopping bags. This was a totally new experience for her. Previously, she would simply have been aware
of others watching her, judging her but certainly not helping her.

And although Robin still had cravings, she learned how to recognize
and cope with them.

"*I won't allow that to happen again. I ask myself am I hungry or is this
a reflection of another problem,*" says Robin about her successful strategy for dealing with temptation.

Learn to ask yourself Robin's question: "Am I eating because I am hungry or for some other reason?"

Robin has taken her weight from 402 pounds down to 217. But it's not just the weight—or maybe even the weight.

"I will never be able to repay what I have received from my fellow TOPS members or even the TOPS organization. YOU SEE, THEY GAVE ME BACK MY LIFE AGAIN," says Robin.

Gave back her life in so many ways. Like being able to give a speech in front of a thousand people and receive a standing ovation. Like being able to tour the region, giving motivational speeches. Like being able to accept compliments graciously. Like going back to college and completing her psychology degree. Like starting graduate school to pursue a career in counseling.

Robin wants to pursue a career helping the severely obese and the terminally ill. Those are both places that Robin knows well. I don't doubt that is what she will do. In finding a group that nurtured her return to the world, Robin also found strength and, above all, hope.

Robin says, "I have found the strength that teaches me that courage is always in me."

Mall Awakening—Janet Andrews

Janet Andrews' self-image had gotten so low that she had given up doing anything about her excess weight. She found her salvation when she reached out to help her nephew and found help from an unexpected source and the hand of fate. This is her story.

When I was about six years old, I started to "blossom" but not like a rose. I became what was called at that time a "chubby girl"—I always hated that word—who had to shop in the special section of the department store for clothes not always in style with what the other kids were wearing.

As we all know, little kids can be cruel. "Fatso" was a name I heard quite often coming from young mouths on the playground, and it was directed at me. I was always the last one to be picked for any game involving teams. Growing up with a weight problem doesn't make you very popular. I withdrew into myself a lot. I wanted desperately to have friends, but I thought all anyone around me was looking at was my excess weight.

When I started junior high school, my family and I moved to a house in a different school district, so I changed schools. I thought in a new school, maybe things in my life would be different, too. I might just find some new friends. But I soon found junior high was just the same old thing with different kids and different teachers. I was still the square peg in the round hole who had also started wearing braces on her teeth.

Beginning to notice boys didn't make things any easier. And believe me, they noticed me, too! I was "fatty-fatty, two-by-four," the one that they laughed at as I walked to and from classes and to my locker each day. Square dancing in PE class was a joke! If I had to dance with a boy, most of them would treat me like I had a dreaded disease and wouldn't hold hands with me unless the teacher made them do it. Even then they'd hold only the very tips of my fingers, distaste on their faces. In their eyes I wasn't pretty, and I wasn't worthy. I was fat, and I was ugly.

High school was filled with dances I never went to. I wasn't asked to go. It was filled with all kinds of sports I either wasn't good at or couldn't participate in due to my excess weight. I did excel at playing the clarinet in the school band, but my teacher never put me in first chair. I was always convinced it was because he was ashamed of the way I looked. There were other, prettier girls he could put in first chair to showcase the band. He even put a boy in that chair—a boy to whom I had taught all the difficult passages. *He* got the solos!

Then there was speech class. I agonized through that semester, sure that every time I got up to give a speech, all anyone could see was my fat. I was positive that they wouldn't be interested in anything I had to say. My knees knocked together, and my voice quavered when I spoke. I was a mess! No one was more surprised than I when I made it through the class with a passing grade!

It would be untrue to say I never had a good day at school. It only seemed the bad days outnumbered the good ones. I truly believe I would never have made it through my childhood and teen years without the support of my family. I always knew I could go home, and I wouldn't be criticized there. They accepted me for who and what I was, and I could be my true self with them. Home became my safe haven, and I had that no matter what the world outside did to me.

I'll admit I carried a pretty big chip on my shoulders. I believed that people should be able to see beyond my fat exterior to the person who lived inside. But I didn't think I had to do anything in particular to help things along. If someone came up and started a conversation with me, I would talk; however, I would never be the one to start the conversation. I thought people had to come to me. If they did, then they must be able to see that I was waiting to be their friend. I think you can guess there weren't many people who fit that bill. Those who did pass the test and break through the barriers I set up became my trusted confidantes, so it was really hard on me when some of them turned out to have a separate agenda and weren't really the friends I thought they were.

Through it all, there was food. Food was my comforter. Food was my crutch. Food was there on the bad days, and food was there on the good days, too. I celebrated with food, and when I was disappointed, frustrated, or angry, food was still there for me.

In the early 70s, after I went through business school and started working as a secretary, I decided that all my problems would be solved if I could just lose my excess weight. I was sure that it was the weight that was holding me back from everything I wanted. So my mom and I decided to "take the bull by the horns" and join Weight Watchers. Both of us did really well with the program, and we both lost all the way to our goal weights. I was finally able to wear all those clothes that I had never been able to wear before. We both looked very slim and trim. So I was sure that popularity would soon follow. Popularity, and maybe even the man of my dreams.

The first thing that I found out was that things didn't change. I was still the same person with the same problems as before. I was still painfully shy with people. And that knight on the white horse—well, he didn't seem to be anywhere around where I was. The second thing I found out was that just because I lost weight, I wasn't able to eat every-thing I wanted to again without putting those pounds right back on. Since I seemed to be failing miserably all the way around, and things weren't going the way I wanted, I just let go of the dreams and let the pounds creep back on. Little by little, a pound at a time, they came back until I had gained every pound I had lost, and then added even more weight to my already expanded frame. After all, my family loved me, skinny or fat. Maybe I didn't need to be thin after all. I retreated back into my shell and hid from the world and from myself. I thor-oughly convinced myself that I would never be thin. I put all thoughts of losing weight out of my mind.

Then, in August of 1995, I heard that Richard Simmons was coming to Seattle. He was going to be at the Southcenter Mall near to where I live. And although I might have given up on seeing a slimmer me, there was someone else in my family who needed Richard's help very badly—my nephew, Jim. I knew that Richard had helped very obese people over the years, and Jim was over six hundred pounds. But would Jim want to go with me to the mall to see Richard? Well, it turned out that he was very interested in going with me.

We had fun trying to exercise with Richard in a crowded mall where everyone kept bumping into each other because we hardly had enough room to breathe, let alone bend and stretch the way he showed us. We listened as Richard extolled the virtues of eating healthy and exercising. And then the line started to form for autographs and the chance to meet Richard in person.

I did something that day that I had rarely ever done. It's something that I would have sworn I didn't have the courage to do. I stood in that line to meet Richard for over an hour. All I knew was that I needed to do it. If Jim was ever going to be helped, I was sure that Richard would be the person to help him. But Jim couldn't stand in a long line. He wasn't able to stand for more than a few minutes at a time without pain and without having difficulty breathing. It would have to be me standing in line, or Jim wouldn't get the chance to meet Richard. So I inched closer and closer, not knowing what I would say when I got up there.

When I finally reached the head of the line, and I was standing in front of Richard, my courage almost failed me. I don't remember my exact words, but I managed to stammer out that my nephew, Jim, really needed his help. He listened to me, never taking his eyes from my face as I turned red with embarrassment, sure that he must think I was a complete idiot. When I'd finished telling him about Jim, his eyes locked with mine, and he simply said, "Janet, it's really great that you care so much about your nephew and his health, but, tell me, what are you doing for YOU?"

I managed to mutter something about planning to do something for me, but that it was Jim that really needed to see him and Jim that needed his help. He smiled very kindly, and he agreed to meet with Jim after the autograph signing was through. True to his word, he did meet with Jim and me a little later. It was funny, but all the time he was talking, I remember thinking, "Why is it that you know me so well? How did you know what I needed to hear?", because Richard's words had struck home, and I knew it was time to do some soul searching.

Was there a "me" worth caring about, worth doing something for? I had hidden myself for so long, I wasn't sure. It all kept coming back to Richard's question: "What are you doing for YOU?" If I was worth caring about, shouldn't I be doing something for me? Maybe it wasn't too late to try and lose some of my own excess weight. I had tried to lose those pounds for everyone and everything else I could think of. Maybe it was time to do it—for ME.

Something else had happened that day. I'm sure none of that day happened by accident. Jim and I not only met Richard, but we also met some ladies who belonged to an organization called TOPS, which met in Burien, right in our own "neck of the woods." Before we left the mall that day, they had invited Jim and me to come to a meeting. A week later, we showed up at our first meeting, and we both decided to join that very evening.

As of January 1, 2001, that was a little over five years and 111 pounds ago. I would love to tell you that losing that 111 pounds was the answer to all of my life's problems. I would love to tell you that the road to my goal has been an easy one. I would really love to tell you that my nephew, Jim, was still on his way to his own weight-loss goal. But I can't do that, because it isn't true.

I still have days when I think I'm not good enough because those feelings of low self-esteem don't ever quite go away. I will continue every day of my life to work on it. There are still days when I don't want to exercise, don't want to eat the right way, and don't want to even hear the word "scale." Yet, the "new improved me" continues to be a fascinating story.

I have learned that I am a "work in progress," and that I am worth doing things for. I have learned that even though I still love food as much as I ever did, I like eating healthier.

Janet does not pretend that she dislikes food. She recognizes that she still loves it, but enjoys being healthier more. Focus on what you are getting, not what you are giving up.

I have learned that the girl who wouldn't lift a finger to exercise will now find time in her schedule to resistance train two to three times a week and do cardio five to six times a week because she feels better when she exercises. I have learned that the scared rabbit who wouldn't think of giving a three-minute speech to a class of teenagers will now get up and teach Sunday School, read scripture in front of her congregation, and run programs for her weight-support group.

TOPS has been my anchor and my support through all of the ups and downs of my weight-loss journey. I have been encouraged by friends to go farther and accomplish things I'd never dreamed I could do, and I will be forever grateful for all the love and support I have received. It has made all the difference.

Family Ties—Stephanie Dellachiara

*Stephanie Dellachiara describes a lifetime of
abusive relationships that increased her weight and crushed her
independence and spirit. It took a baby and the promise of
renewed family relationships to reverse her self-image, her
weight, and her physical ailments.*

I have never, yes never, known what it feels like to be slim. During my childhood and teen years, my mother told me I was fat. She sewed all my clothes and always complained that she had to use extra-large patterns. She was five feet tall and weighed between 110 and 113 pounds her entire adult life.

I look back at pictures of myself and am amazed when I see a lovely, slim, young girl and teenager. When I told my mother about compliments people gave me, she would tell me they were lying to not hurt my feelings, but *she* was telling me the truth. Even on my wedding day, she was angry because I ruined the look of the dress. I was five foot, six inches, and weighed 125 pounds. The dress was plain empire waist, like an hourglass and, hey, I look at the pictures now, and I was beautiful. But then I felt ugly. It is at times like these that I thank God she is not my birth mother—I was adopted.

Anyway, I never felt good about myself. I lived in an abusive house as a child. I married an abusive husband. I was always told everything was my fault. So I was beaten emotionally and physically from the outside, and since that was all I knew, I beat myself emotionally and physically from the inside.

I was afraid of everyone, especially authority figures. My "mother" fit the role of the main character in *Mommy Dearest*, even to cleaning the tile floor with the toothbrush. I would come home from school and find all my clothes from my closet on the floor, the mattress pulled off the bed, the drawers on top of the bureau—even the desk emptied—all because I had hung a blouse in the wrong section or not dry mopped under the bed and had missed a "planted" wad of dust. *I* would be responsible for breaking the hairbrushes when she would start hitting me with them because I made her so angry. Even today, I have no idea what I did wrong.

I was very quiet and withdrawn in school. One of my teachers saw some potential and put me on the yearbook staff. I was a sophomore and had to go to the freshmen homerooms and give a speech about selling ads to raise money to print the yearbook. I liked doing it. On the yearbook staff I felt I belonged, that I was part of something. In my junior year I was made co-editor with a senior. WOW! When we went with the newspaper staff to a Journalism Day at UCLA, we were assigned to cars. I went with some seniors and had the most wonderful day of my life. When I got home, my mother asked for the name of the parent who drove the car I was in. I had to tell her I went with a senior. You see, I was not allowed to ride with other kids. But I was told by my teacher, an authority figure, to ride in that car. Damned if I do, and, as I thought, damned if I don't. So, first my mother went and reamed out the teacher and then came back and beat the living tar out of me. She also insisted that I be taken off the yearbook staff. She would be in jail if I were a kid today. But, it was still the most wonderful day of my life.

The teacher did not remove me from the staff but instead had me do my work during lunch and recess. At the end of the year when the yearbooks came out, I was listed as staff and got more punishment.

So my self-image was poor. I had no dates. My senior year my mother put me in a dance class. I met a guy, Gerry, from our basketball team, and we learned to waltz and hop together but when prom time came, no one asked me. On prom night, three other girls and I went to a movie. I was sure I was not asked because I was too fat, and I was certain no one wanted to be seen with me. Thirty years later, my mother told me and my daughters that my friend, Gerry, had indeed asked to take me to the prom, but she had told him no. When I asked why, she just said I must have been grounded or something—she could not remember. Years later, I had occasion to meet a few of my former teachers, and they all said the same thing—I was a *thin and sickly* child. Not fat, as I thought, but thin and sickly!

After graduation, I was fortunate to go away to a private college. I thought I would belong, like I did on the yearbook staff, but I did not. I felt completely anonymous. Instead of growing, I withdrew. The meals were cafeteria style, and I started slowly gaining weight. I blended into a routine of working and going to class. During that time, my parents moved to a new house. After three years of school, I developed a medical problem that interfered with my continuation at school. I needed to return home for a while. When my parents moved, they did not set up a room for me in their new house, and there was not a single thing in their home that showed I even existed. They had to rent a cot so I could have something to sleep on. My mother was so angry with me for complicating her life. I had gained thirty pounds, and I was ordered to get them off and not allowed any more than nine hundred calories a day. She was embarrassed to be seen with me.

I had completed three years of college, so I wanted to continue, but I had come home and now they would not help pay, so I went to work in St. Francis Hospital in Lynwood. It was June 1964. I did not want to date, but my mother forced me to join a young adults club at a church near the hospital. I participated in some of the group activities, and that seemed to satisfy her. I soon became co-president and editor of the newsletter. We won an award for our newsletter. I represented our club as girl of the year, and I started feeling like a Real Person. People liked me, and I liked me. My soon-to-be husband was a member, and we started dating. He treated me with respect. No one had treated me like that in all my life. I would get ready for a date and look in the mirror and can remember smiling and feeling good.

Of course, I was a perfectionist, so my work at the hospital was good, and I was transferred to the Intensive Care Unit. A doctor thought so much of my work, he wanted to sponsor me through medical school, but my mother put a stop to that. No child of hers was going to receive charity. I did change jobs, but I didn't go back to school—I got married instead.

Later, my husband told me that his brother had bet him that he could not get someone like me to marry him. He had dated me, proposed to me, and married me all on a bet. The man was psychotic. He made me pay every day of our marriage. According to him, the marriage license meant he owned me. I was worthless. I was not part of the family. I was ugly, lazy, and fat.

Gone was the co-president, newsletter editor, happy, smiling, girl of the year. Back was someone who was slapped down and smothered, silenced in horror, buried, and eventually covered with weight.

I had two wonderful children but a miserable marriage. Things only got worse when I was pregnant again, and my husband ordered me to have an abortion. I refused and left. My parents told me I was wrong. Of course, I did as I was told and returned to him although I did not get an abortion. I almost lost my baby, but didn't. I stayed married for six more years. My weight was over two hundred pounds.

I believe my life began when I eventually divorced my husband in 1981. I went to work for a group of doctors. I was independent for the first time. I had to learn what that really meant. But I started off with a handicap.

That same year I was diagnosed with diabetes. The physicians prescribed Mysoline, but I never got any nutritional advice except to stay away from sweets. So my weight did not move much. It was only three years later when I changed my job and met another physician that I got good nutritional advice. I lost some weight, but my weight was cycling. My life was spent working and raising my three daughters alone (fourteen, ten, and six when I divorced), slowly building a life for myself. Still fat.

In May 1991, I took a local position with a medical billing company. My girls, Michelle, Kristie, and Jamie were growing up, but I still wasn't doing anything about my weight. I guess I didn't care much about me; there didn't seem to be time.

I was unbelievably self-conscious. When I would go out with friends to a restaurant, I would never order big meals or dessert because I was sure the waitress was thinking I was too fat. I always wore loose-fitting clothes. I felt self-conscious in the market if I had cookies or ice cream in the wagon. I thought people were looking at me, and I'm sure they were thinking that I should not buy those things. So when I got to the checkout counter, I'd tell the cashier that my kids were having a slumber party, as if she cared. Then when I got home I'd eat everything.

And that's the way it stayed until December 1996, when I saw my granddaughter take her first breath. After about half an hour, her mom and dad finally let me hold her. It was then that I knew I had made the COMMITMENT. I had a choice: Did I want to be a picture in the album and have my daughter say, "This is a picture of my mommy; she died before you were old enough to know her?" Or, did I want to sit with her and say, "This is a picture of your mommy wearing my shoes and necklaces and playing dress up just like you do." Did I want to know and love her and have her know and love me? YES!

The feeling of holding her was overwhelmingly positive. I can't really describe it. I had so many negative relationships in my life, but this baby was going to be a positive influence, not just on my relationship with her and the other members of my family, but also perhaps most of all with myself.

So I went back to my doctor.

I went to a diabetes education class. I followed the Exchange System. I lost forty pounds; then I hit a wall. I found a group that met on Monday nights so that I could go after work. I joined November 17, 1997. I felt welcome; I received encouragement and inspiration. I belonged. I started to lose weight and get my diabetes under control.

Terrific Tactic

Use the Exchange System, the best form of nutritional guidance and the system on which virtually every worthwhile weight-loss program is based.

I found that measuring out every portion size was really critical for me. It is too easy to underestimate. Oh, it looks like a cup, but it actually is a cup and a half. *I would always make sure that the scales were out in the kitchen so I couldn't cop out of weighing foods.* I continued to lose, using the Exchange System and by setting small, attainable goals. *With my history of low self-esteem, I did not want to set myself up for failure.*

Terrific Tactic

Keep the food scales easily available in the kitchen so that there's no excuse not to use them.

That's not the end of my story, however. In May 1998, I was found unconscious at my desk. The paramedics took me to the Emergency Room, and I then spent three days in Intensive Care. Diagnosis—epilepsy. Life knocked out from under me. Driver's license taken away, cannot be left alone with my granddaughter, don't take a shower when no one is home. At work, I started experiencing seizures daily, became situationally depressed, and was put on Zoloft, which helped, but the seizures kept increasing. Finally by October, I was declared unable to work and put on disability. Stuck at home—just me, my refrigerator, and my fork.

It is at times of crisis that you need positive people in your life. I still belonged to TOPS, and in spite of all that had been happening, I had lost another ten pounds. I knew that if I turned to food to "comfort" me I would destroy what I had accomplished and further endanger my physical health. So I told my group I needed help. They were great.

When I was no longer allowed to drive, the ladies in our chapter took turns driving me around. Our weight recorder, Betty Keylon, is one of the most inspirational people I know. She really seems to understand all of our behaviors. There is always an encouragement, an enlightenment— "Do you realize you seem to...?" "Are you ill?" "You are dropping weight faster than is sensible," etc.

When I was first diagnosed with epilepsy and getting so anxious and also depressed, she just kept telling me to stay calm, I would get through it, I was strong, everyone cared.

That is exactly what I needed to hear. When I was home alone, scared and looking in the refrigerator, I remembered her words and would get water or have some broth or tea instead of just whatever fit in my mouth.

And that's how I made it.

In December of that year, I reached my goal weight.

I have made myself active. I am co-leader of my chapter. I write a monthly newsletter. I get games and contests going. I try to give imaginative programs complete with music, audience participation, and meaningful inspiration. I speak at the Diabetes Education Classes at the hospital, telling them about how I have been helped to lose the needed weight and get my diabetes under control.

Now I do not care who sees me eat what and what is in my wagon. Actually, I don't buy junk food anymore. I do get dessert in the restaurant sometimes and enjoy it, but I can order anything I wish without feeling self-conscious. In fact, I can do anything I wish now without feeling self-conscious. The sense of family brought about by the arrival of my granddaughter and my weight-loss group have made all the difference.

If you judge people you have no time to love them. – Mother Theresa

Guardian Angels—Vanessa Netherlain

Vanessa Netherlain describes how self-esteem and weight are linked to relationships. At critical times in her life, she had positive influences that minimized the damage of the detrimental ones. Eventually, she reversed her weight and self-image by learning to take responsibility for eliminating the negative relationships and fostering the positive ones. In so doing, she found the courage to realize her dreams.

Do you believe in guardian angels? I think they take many forms, and I want to tell you about mine. In my roller-coaster life, they have been there just when I needed them to pick me up and set me straight again.

I was not a fat child, but not thin. My family always pushed me to go outside and play; otherwise I would have been huge. I was blessed with a love of food and a slow metabolism. My grandmother and her side of the family were all obese. In fact, I have a couple of great aunts and uncles who are over 450 pounds. I always thought that my mother was lucky; she was always thin, but I found out later from my grandfather that she also battled her weight by starving herself.

My grandparents used to take me on weekend trips up and down the California coast, and my favorite part was that I got to eat out at every meal. I remember my grandfather always telling me my middle name was, "I'm Hungry." When most kids would complain about having to come inside to eat lunch or dinner, I was already at the door asking how soon it would be ready. My grandmother was an incredible cook who made all kinds of wonderful things: chicken dumplings, pies, breads, cookies, and cakes. One of my family mottoes was, "What's full got to do with it?"

Despite this I didn't gain any significant weight until adolescence.

No, not just because of adolescence; there were other things going on in my life that I see now had a huge impact on me.

My mom and dad divorced when I was a baby, and I never knew my father. My mom was desperately trying to make it on her own, but she was not always successful. We would go back and forth between some rental house and my grandparents' home, where I would spend virtually all of my available free time. When I was eight, my mother got involved with a man and eventually married him. He turned out to be a heroin addict and a thief who stole money from my mom who would then have to call my grandparents, as she had nothing to feed me. Fortunately for me, he spent a lot of time in prison. Thank God for my grandparents. I had stability at their house. The cupboards were full of food.

When I was thirteen, I left my mom and went to live with my grandparents permanently. They had been my angels, and now they were my guardians. Soon after, my mom moved to Northern California with her new boyfriend—another loser who was an alcoholic. A year later my mom called my grandparents from New Mexico and asked them to wire her money for the bus trip home. They wired the money, and we went to the bus stop to meet her. We waited and waited. She never showed. (She never showed again. Years later, when I was twenty-two, a police officer came to the door and told me my mother had been found. She had died of an overdose in the back of one of her friend's pickup trucks.)

At the time my mother was a no-show at the bus stop, my grandmother had just been diagnosed with leukemia. She survived another year and died when I was fifteen. During these two years I had gained thirty pounds. The summer between my tenth and eleventh grade I decided I was going to get thin. The demands of high school are pretty tough, especially in California, where there is a lot of pressure to be one of the "beautiful people." Without my mom or grandmother around to guide me, I went on a starvation diet. I had to hide it from my grandfather and would say I had eaten a sandwich or something before he got home from work. I am grateful to him, however, because when he realized what I was doing, he would get up early and make me a full hot breakfast in the mornings. This is from a man who hates to cook. What an angel.

I had dropped thirty pounds by starving myself and managed to keep the weight off by joining the swim team until senior year, when I quit. I had met my husband-to-be and decided to make my last year "easy" since I already had racked up most of my college-prep credits. Then, after graduation, I moved in with my boyfriend at the age of eighteen, and I was married at nineteen. Biggest mistake of my life. My weight went up and up.

My ex-husband liked thin women and didn't hesitate to tell me. He was very selfish and demanding. I am a redhead, but he was always bugging me to dye my hair blonde. He was famous for telling me how much he wanted me to be skinny. We would fight about it, and then he would get a pizza and ask me to eat it with him. Then he would tell me how much my body repulsed him. His words cut me like a knife. I was with him for eighteen months, and he drove my self-esteem into the ground. He told me how fat and ugly I was. Of course, this did nothing to inspire me—just the opposite. Food became my best friend. Food didn't put me down; food was always there for me. As I continued to put on weight, he continued to emotionally abuse me. Eventually, I weighed more than two hundred pounds.

I started to stay away as much as possible. After he lost his job, he started staying in the garage all night "building up his contracting business." Yeah, right. He was doing drugs. One day I woke up, drove to his friend's house, and told him I would not stay married to a drug user. Putting up with emotional abuse was one thing; putting up with drugs was another. So we divorced. Shortly after, my so-called "best friend" told me she had slept with him and suspected there had been many others. Thank God, I got him out of my life.

Without him around telling me how horrible I was, I started to take care of myself again. A friend of mine said that I "blossomed" when I left him. I got excited about life again, starting to take care of myself and my appearance. Eventually, I began dating again and was amazed that men found me attractive. Now, I had to do something about that weight.

Unfortunately, I did not know how to diet. I had always thought that to lose weight, you had to stop eating. So I did. I had starved off that thirty pounds in just a few short weeks in high school. Then a friend (who must have been an angel in disguise) introduced me to TOPS. It was July 1992 in San Bernardino. I started to learn about eating sensibly, drinking water, and exercising. The friendship I found was priceless and the support, invaluable.

In September of 1992, I decided that moving to Myrtle Creek, Oregon, would be a good choice for me to start my life again. I found a wonderful chapter in a nearby town called Winston, and they helped me to take off an additional twenty pounds. Unfortunately, I found that I had to move back to California four months later. After I arrived back in California everyone I knew complimented me on my weight loss. I became overconfident and decided that I did not need a weight-loss support group anymore. I only had ten more pounds to lose, and I could do it myself. Boy, was I wrong. By 1994, I had put half my weight back on.

Enter a new angel and positive influence par excellence, Mark, the new love of my life who cared enough about me to suggest in just the right way that I return to TOPS. With my friends at TOPS and Mark's support, I lost the weight I had put on, and was again ten pounds from my goal. I was stuck at this weight for almost a year. My life had gotten busy, and I was not working very hard at it. I have a bad habit of losing my momentum every so often.

In March 1996, I began to put on weight and was not sure why. The next month, I found out that I was pregnant. "Oh no," I thought. "All that work for nothing!" I did try to keep my weight under control, but it didn't work. I worked full time and had no time for exercise. Not to mention I was constantly hungry!

On August 10, 1996, I married Mark. We had our ceremony on horseback. It was wonderful! I rode my horse sidesaddle, and all the guests sat on hay bales. We then moved to Harvard, Illinois, when Mark got a job with Motorola. I had my son on December 20, 1996. It was a wonderful time for me.

I guess you could say I had "made the connection," as Oprah says. For the first time, I kept a food chart. The chapter charged us fifty cents if we didn't, and I was too cheap to pay it. I can't tell you how much this helped me. I realized how much I was actually eating, even though I thought I was "being good." I also made exercise a regular part of my day. It's so important. I know it's hard work, but every bit worth the effort!

Terrific Tactic

Vanessa makes some type of exercise a regular part of her day.

By the time my husband was transferred to Texas in November 1997, I had lost over fifty pounds.

On April 22, 1998, I reached my goal. It was such a great feeling to achieve something that I had been trying to do for six years plus. Now I feel I can do anything. It's amazing what TOPS has done for me, not just in losing weight but also in lots of areas of my life. Recently, I participated in a skit at Fun Day in San Antonio. This was a big step for me since I have always had a fear of speaking in front of people, and this skit involved not only being on stage by myself but also adlibbing! I was scared, but I can't tell you how good I felt afterward!

I have so much self-confidence and self-esteem now. Overweight people are very conscious of the fat on their bodies and feel like everyone is looking and thinking, "What is that fat lady doing here?" It makes getting involved in life a very scary experience. When I reached my goal weight, I felt like I could do anything. I am dying to start trying new things like scuba diving, mountain climbing, learning to fly an airplane, etc. I used to be so shy; now I have done programs, skits, and was even leader for a year. Of course, some things will have to wait until my six-month-old baby is a bit older, of course. ...

I have come to realize that "nothing tastes as good as thin feels." Maintaining my weight is not easy with two small boys and a husband. But I try to balance my eating. If I overdo on some days—especially the weekends when my husband is off and we go out to eat—then I try to cut back on other days and exercise.

T e r r i f i c   T a c t i c

If Vanessa gets a little off track with her program she doesn't get discouraged; she merely makes adjustments and sensible compensations,
the key to sensible lifestyle change.

I also subscribe to magazines like *Shape* and *Fitness*, to keep me focused and to get ideas on exercise and eating. Most of all, though, I make sure to surround myself with positive people. Those guardian angels didn't just love me and protect me; they guided me to do the right things. Without those angels, I know I would not be where I am today.

> *It is far better to be alone than in bad company.*
> *– George Washington*

I'm Not Afraid to Live My Dreams—Nancy Best

*Nancy Best reminds us that it takes courage to face the difficulty
of reality but that when we do
we can surprise ourselves.*

I could never do that! Ride a bike, walk on stilts, parallel park a car? But I did! Sure, I fell a few times, had many skinned knees, bumped a few cars, but with encouragement and the advice of a good coach, I persevered and accomplished all of these feats.

I am capable of achieving and doing great things. How much of this capability I use depends on my identity. As an outgoing, cheerful, energetic person, I realize I must tap into my resources to match my identity. What is the one thing missing in my identity? CONSISTENCY!

If I begin to question who I am, I have pulled the rug from under my feet. If I don't know who I am, how can I decide what to do?

What am I afraid of? Making a mistake, making the wrong choice, worried that I may not be good enough? Afraid of succeeding? The choice is mine. I do not want to be paralyzed by fear.

All of my accomplishments happen when I take the first step. Not a large step; a baby step will do. In fact, small steps will get me to my dream. And, one day I will realize I am there!

I have so many people who love me, support me, and cheer me on as I move toward my dreams. I am grateful for them. The road to a goal is a lonely road. Reach out, my friend, and take my hand. We're almost there! When I ask for directions, I will seek those who have traveled this road with a map.

Living my dreams is a journey. It builds character. There will always be times when I wonder if I have what it takes to fulfill my dreams or even if I deserve them. Fear is a normal part of human nature, and I can accept that fear will occur during the process of striving for my goal. The only way to get past this fear is to go through it, not around it. I can do it!

What am I waiting for? I know there are no guarantees, but the rewards are plentiful because I believe in myself. It's up to me to create my own life, and I will create one that is filled with dreams. *I'm not afraid to live my dreams!*

Rankin's Reminders

Lens Restorers

Find a positive support group. Self-esteem can only be improved through positive interaction with others.

Remove yourself from the company of negative, judgmental people. They will hook your self-doubt and sense of inadequacy and bring you down.

Don't set yourself up for failure. You are primed to jump to negative conclusions about yourself. Set small, attainable goals, and focus on the short term. Think about losing the next pound, not the next fifty.

Be aware of those critical internal tapes. Listen to how you are talking to yourself. Be compassionate with yourself.

Eliminate extreme words like "always" and "never," as well as obligation words like "ought" and "should," from your vocabulary.

Analyze hunger. Your thoughts aren't always what they seem to be either; neither is hunger.

Have courage. Nancy Best reminds us that fear is natural but cannot be allowed to stop you.

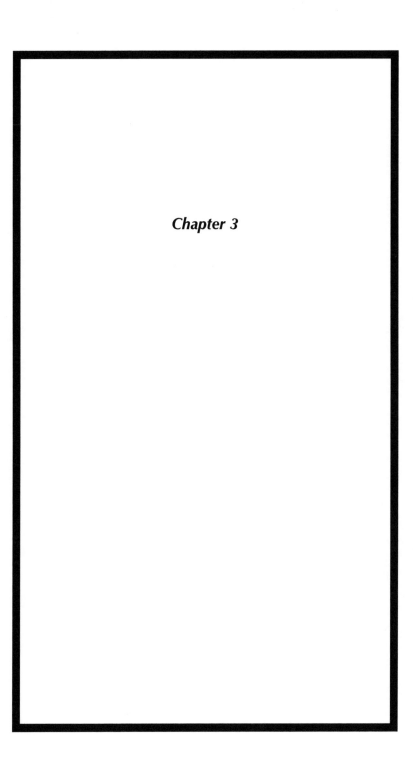

Chapter 3

The Choice of Positive Thinking

Adopt the right mental attitude

> *Consult not your fears but your hopes and dreams. Think not about your frustrations but about your unfulfilled potential. Concern yourself not with what you have tried and failed but what is still possible for you. – Pope John XXIII*

The abilities to control the mind, direct consciousness, and manage emotions are the greatest powers that human beings possess. But these skills don't happen naturally. They need to be trained, developed, and honed. They require effort. Positive thinking is a choice.

Positive thinking has many advantages. Research shows that those who practice it live considerably longer than those who don't. Positive thinkers are assumed to have less disease risk and higher recovery rates when they do get sick. One study showed that successful people have twice as many positive thoughts as negative thoughts.

There are misconceptions about positive thinking, however. Being positive does not mean constantly wearing a smile and feeling good. Positive thinking does not require the perception that the world is a wonderful place and nothing bad can ever happen.

Positive thinking does not require the perception that the world is a wonderful place and nothing bad can ever happen.

The phrase, positive thinking, is a misnomer. A more accurate expression might be *adaptive thinking*. The fact is that difficult life situations do occur. Unexpected challenges and obstacles frequently appear.

The value of adaptive thinking is not in denying the seriousness of these difficulties, ignoring them, or pretending that they don't exist. The value in adaptive thinking is coping with adversity so that effective action is possible. Many life events are extremely difficult and potentially very depressing. It is understandable and natural for anyone given a cancer diagnosis, for example, to feel depressed and defeated. But such a response, while understandable and logical, is not very *adaptive*. It is likely to prevent effective action. It is likely to become a negative, self-fulfilling prophecy.

So what characteristics of adaptive thinking make it effective?

Adaptive thinking allows for the setting and effective pursuit of positive goals. Adaptive thinking allows for creating positive solutions to problems. Adaptive thinking decreases negative moods. Adaptive thinking increases energy.

The anticipation of difficult situations is helpful if it leads to effective planning, but most of the time it leads to unproductive worrying. Worrying is not only a waste of time but a waste of energy, too. Anxiety and worry translate into cellular activity that can drain energy and affect behavior. Energy is a key component in weight loss. Energy needs to be maintained at a high level. When energy sinks, several unwanted results occur. Hunger and fatigue increase. You are less likely to exercise, make good food choices, and pay attention to behavior.

An adaptive attitude will lead to the birth and execution of positive goals. Mental activity is more than just words, though. Images are more important than words. The visual system is older, more primitive, and thus more powerful than words or even logic. Putting positive images into the mind is a powerful way of realizing goals. Even when the message is verbal, it is almost always translated into an image. In the first story in this chapter, Richard Willoughby, trying to recover from a knife attack, describes how he used a simple mantra—"I refuse to be a cripple"—to focus on his goal. Admittedly, it would have been ideal to state his mantra in more positive terms—for example, "I will walk again"—but nonetheless his words conjured for him not just a message of defiance but also an image of mobility and recovery.

Because images work in the subconscious, they have tremendous power. Negative images can be like computer viruses attacking the hard drive—in this case, your head. Positive images generate motivation, and they impact mood. As I have described in the chapter on the mind-body connection, positive mental states translate into healthier bodies. It's as if positive images recharge cellular batteries. It is no surprise then to learn that many of the successful people featured in this book used visualization in their arsenal of effective weapons.

Adaptive thinking involves overcoming fear—the fear that you won't succeed; the fear that success can't be maintained; the fear that the other shoe is about to drop. Life does throw obstacles in the way of your best plans and can hook these anxieties and send you spiraling down. Staying focused on goals rather than being distracted by the obstacles is the key to adaptive thinking.

> *Obstacles are those frightful things you see when you take your eyes off your goal. – Henry Ford*

A positive attitude also means letting go of anxieties and especially the fear of uncertainty. We all want as much control as possible. The search and drive for that control is one of the major causes of stress. However, control is often illusory. We would be far better off embracing uncertainty rather than fruitlessly trying to manage it. When we can let go of that fear, wonderful things can happen.

The Maine Man—Richard Willoughby

Richard Willoughby's story highlights the difference between the popular fantasy of positive thinking and the reality of adaptive thinking. When it mattered most—when faced with paralysis, obesity, and relapse—Richard's adaptive thinking allowed him to progress rather than remain stuck or even slip back.

No backbone. No one had ever accused Richard Willoughby of being spineless. Yet, when I saw him for the first time, rocking gently to the jukebox music coming from the bar on the twenty-fifth floor of the Galt House Hotel in Louisville, Kentucky, I had no idea that backbone was such a large part of this man's amazing story.

Richard Willoughby is the Maine Man. Standing at nearly six feet, five inches tall, he cuts an imposing figure at the best of times. Now that he can stand up straight, that is.

Richard has always been big. In high school, he weighed 250 pounds. His weight was evenly distributed about his big body but particularly about his belly. Even then, he did not consider himself obese.

By the time Richard owned a restaurant and nightclub, he weighed 380 pounds, but that still didn't bother him. Life was about to change for Richard—and it had nothing to do with his weight.

One night in February 1992, Richard was working at his nightclub when there was a disturbance. Richard took matters into his own hands and confronted the offender, then began to remove him from the club. Rather than take the man out through the front of the club, Richard decided to take him out the back way, through the kitchen. On the way through the kitchen, the drunk offender broke loose and, grabbing a large butcher's knife, plunged it six inches into Richard's neck.

Richard was rushed to the emergency room where it took surgeons several hours to remove the knife and repair the wound as best they could. Richard's vertebrae had been cut and his spinal chord nearly severed.

It was awhile before Richard was conscious of anything at all, let alone the seriousness of his plight. He was physically and mentally numb. Once he recovered from the anesthesia of the procedure, Richard gradually became aware of memories of the event and feelings of anger. Problem was, he still couldn't feel anything physically. He was paralyzed from all points south of his neck.

The doctors were brutally honest with Richard. He would never walk again. He wouldn't be able to use his arms either. He was paralyzed for life. Three hundred and eighty pounds condemned to life in a wheelchair. Almost a complete vegetable. This didn't sit well with Richard—he really didn't like vegetables so that the prospect of being one was not at all palatable.

And Richard is nothing if not independent. He reacted completely in character. What went through Richard's mind, almost immediately, was soon to become his mantra: "I refuse to be a cripple."

In the weeks and days that followed there was a significant battle for Richard's mind. Each day he would arrange for a sign to be put at the end of his bed that simply stated his mantra—"I refuse to be a cripple." Each day his doctors ordered the sign to be removed. They did not want Richard living in fantasy. The sooner he accepted his fate, the quicker he could adjust to life as a paraplegic. Fat chance. Each time the sign was taken down—on doctor's orders—Richard, somehow, got it put back up.

Richard simply was not ready to accept being a quadriplegic yet—if ever.

"I can't live this way."

Richard couldn't be a quadriplegic—he had his fourteen-year-old daughter to raise. If nothing else, he owed it to her to be able to move. His daughter and mother were there at his bedside every day—putting up that sign, reinforcing his resolve, and shoring up the fantasy of movement against that ghastly specter of paralysis.

Another occasional visitor was the preacher, who lent his force to the effort for Richard's mind by giving some practical advice.

"Stop asking why; ask instead what you can do," the preacher reinforced. Richard responded. Perhaps he could will himself to move. But how do you will yourself out of paralysis?

Richard had been trying to will his paralyzed muscles to move. It seemed some sort of psychic experiment, like bending spoons or making objects move with just the power of thought. Despite the fact that this particular psychic experiment had yet to work, Richard *knew* that there must be a way of regaining feeling and movement.

"If I just try a little harder," he thought.

Then it happened. One morning Richard felt something. A tingling sensation in his leg. More, a spasm. Yes, a spasm! One small spasm in the foot, but one great leap in the imagination. The spasm wasn't just a spasm; it was a sign for Richard that progress wasn't beyond reach. It transformed hope into tangible progress. He was right: he could recover!

"If I just thought hard enough, I knew I could create a muscle spasm," Richard recalls.

Yes, Richard could create a spasm, especially when he was looking at that sign. I REFUSE TO BE A CRIPPLE.

Each day, Richard worked with the therapist a bit longer and a bit harder than was scheduled. Each day there was progress. By the time Richard left the hospital a few months later, he had regained some sensation and a little mobility but was still condemned to a wheelchair. The tough part was about to come. On the upside, Richard had lost twenty pounds. As depressing as his prospects were, Richard knew his salvation depended on his attitude.

"I made a conscious decision to be positive."

It's a good thing that Richard made a conscious decision to be positive, because there wasn't a whole lot to be positive about unconsciously. You can tell yourself that things could be worse, but when you're in a wheelchair, have a fourteen-year-old daughter, and live on the second floor, it doesn't really feel as if things could be much worse. Richard knew it was going to be tough—very tough.

"*I was scared to come home*," says Richard. Home. No around-the-clock nursing. No meals. No doctors to fight. No one telling him to bring down that sign. Yes, a therapist came regularly, but progress was painfully slow. Richard was no closer to getting out of that wheelchair. He was severely depressed.

One incident stands as a milestone in Richard's journey the wrong way up the street of hope. An avid NASCAR fan, Richard had gone to the Talladega 500, a major race held in Alabama each year, several times before, and he decided to do it again—even if he was in a wheelchair. So arrangements were made for Richard to attend the race in 1992. The attempt to raise his spirits with this trip backfired as badly as a car limping into the pits with engine trouble.

First, it seemed to take forever to get prepared for the trip. It seemed to be taking an army of people to gather personal belongings and make the most basic of preparations. The long trip in a friend's van was interminable. Getting to and from the track was agonizingly slow. Then there was the race itself. Watching cars streak past at breakneck speed at the height of mobility only made Richard more aware of his own broken neck and complete immobility. In the end, the whole experience was not the lift that had been intended.

"I saw how much work it was for everyone to get me there and take care of me. It really depressed me," recalls Richard.

Yes, depression, the refuge of those with difficult life situations. For two long years Richard struggled, making small strides that were metaphorical rather than literal. He rarely got out of the wheelchair or out of his house. His frustration was growing. His helplessness was growing. His waistline was growing.

Up to this point, Richard had entrusted the complete care of his business to a valued friend and employee, Scott. Now Scott was about to repay Richard's trust in a way that he could never have imagined. Concerned about Richard's declining mental state and increasing physical size, Scott suggested that Richard attend the local TOPS group's meeting. Scott had several family members who attended TOPS with good results.

So in the fall of 1994 Richard decided to attend the local TOPS group meeting. Richard was apprehensive merely about leaving the house, so that the idea of going to a TOPS meeting filled him with apprehension. For one thing, Richard had stopped weighing himself after he passed three hundred pounds, and he thought he must be close to 450 by now. Imagine his embarrassment, then, when at his first TOPS meeting on a chilly November evening, he topped the scales at 515 pounds.

Richard didn't say much at that first meeting where there were about thirty people in attendance. He chose to sit in the background and observe. Several important things happened at that first meeting, however.

"I was really amazed how kind everyone at TOPS was on that first occasion," recalls Richard. Receiving only encouragement was very big for this big man. For two years, he had been soldiering almost entirely on his own. Actually, he had been doing that his whole life. But now, to go public and get such overwhelming support was a significant turning point. Not one person at that meeting did anything to reinforce Richard's embarrassment. Everyone made him feel he could lose the weight. Everyone. Richard also found out how much he weighed and was embarrassed.

"I knew I would have to tell people who asked how much I weighed," he recalls.

Embarrassment may be uncomfortable, but it is Nature's motivator. Richard vowed to make every attempt to reduce his weight. He also had to repay the faith that all of the TOPS members had in him.

There was one other crucial aspect about that first TOPS meeting. Richard had been working overtime on his physical therapy and had reached the point where he could shuffle along with support, albeit with great difficulty. For the first time, at that first TOPS meeting, Richard went public without his wheelchair. In fact, he never took his wheelchair to TOPS. Ever.

By the end of 1994 Richard had lost twenty pounds. A few months later he had lost another forty, getting him closer to where he thought he was before that first TOPS meeting.

Tuesday nights were TOPS meetings, and they became an important part of Richard's recovery. But it didn't seem enough.

"I would go to the meetings on Tuesday and be fired up for a few days, but by Friday I was beginning to slip again," says Richard.

And it showed. By the end of 1995 Richard had regained the sixty pounds he had lost.

Richard knows that persistence is the key to success. So at the beginning of 1996 he resolved again to lose weight.

"I was determined never to be here again," Richard said of the five-hundred-plus point he now found himself reluctantly revisiting on the scale. This time around he made an even greater commitment. "I realized that I needed to be more involved," he admits.

This perception led him to make a momentous decision. If he was going to commit himself completely, he couldn't also be running a business. So he sold it.

Throwing himself into his mission to save himself, Richard now became the co-leader of the TOPS group. This involved him in new activities, like leading group discussions and spending more time at outside workshops that met quarterly. Richard put himself deliberately in this position so that he would feel the added pressure of having to be a good example as a group leader.

In this second time around, Richard was forced on by more than just his own determination. The TOPS leader kept pushing him by setting small but manageable goals. "She was a bit pushy, but it was what I needed," he says.

Behavioral scientists fond of jargon call it "proximal goal-setting"; the average person in the street calls it "taking one day at a time." Whatever you call it, small, manageable goals are one of the secrets to successful weight loss. Richard, with help from his leader, resolved to lose twenty pounds between each quarterly workshop. Not only did Richard achieve this, but he also recorded the single biggest weight loss.

Terrific Tactic

Set small, manageable, behavioral goals.

As the weight dropped off, Richard was able to begin and maintain a better exercise regimen that benefited his mobility as well as his weight. The overall effect of this rededication of himself to himself was a consistent and maintained commitment.

"I said my TOPS pledge every single day, like prayers," says Richard. It was now an everyday commitment that stretched seven days a week, not the three or four it had in the previous year. "I was on my program seven days a week."

It wasn't just inner strength and an adaptive attitude that kept Richard focused. There were significant others. First, there were the TOPS members who had been so instrumental in making Richard feel so welcome at that initial meeting. As well as seeing them at the Tuesday night meetings, Richard would call them on a regular basis— as a friend rather than a TOPS member.

There wasn't a need to talk about TOPS. That group had given birth to friendships that were self-sustaining. These conversations reinforced the idea that losing weight was really a smaller part of regaining control of life in general. There was no need for a running commentary on weight loss. Friendship and support transcend the scales.

Then there was Richard's daughter. When he was lying motionless in the hospital, it was the thought of his daughter that kept Richard from giving up. He didn't want to be a paralyzed father. She would come and simply sit by his bedside for hours at a time—every day. And once he was out of the hospital and in the TOPS program, his daughter was just as necessary for Richard's resolve.

One evening, Richard returned from a TOPS meeting, happy with a five-pound weight loss. He was feeling hungry and started to rummage around in the kitchen. He came across some chips that his daughter had stashed at the back of the closet. Richard had just opened the bag when he heard a voice.

"What do you think you're doing?" asked his daughter.

"Hey, I lost five pounds last week; give me some slack," said Richard.

"Yes, well, we don't want you *gaining* five pounds this week," said his daughter, grabbing the chips from his hand.

Richard was absorbing this chiding when he heard a strange rustling sound from the kitchen. He went to explore and found his daughter removing all of her less than low-fat snacks.

"I can see that if I'm going to help you, I can't have this food around," she said, tossing most of it away in the garbage and taking the rest to the relative privacy of her own room.

Then there was the TOPS membership in general. By the end of 1996 Richard had lost ninety-seven pounds, earning him the title, "Mr. Inspiration." In this role he visited TOPS groups and told his story to motivate others.

"The speaking helped me stay on track. After all, I felt as if the whole state was riding on me."

Then there was his mother. She called every Tuesday to find out how Richard had done during the previous week. She was never critical, always encouraging. Perhaps that is where Richard got his strong inner voice—the one that refused to be beaten.

By the end of 1997 Richard had lost another ninety-one pounds. His mobility was returning. It wasn't just TOPS events that he could go to without a wheelchair. During this time he started those daily tasks that most of us take for granted. Like driving.

"I was really scared to take the wheel at first. But then it was really unbelievable," Richard recalls.

Unbelievable to be free. To sit in a vehicle that had wheels and to feel it was a passport not a prison. Other activities were incredibly liberating. Like bending down to tie his own shoes. Riding a bike. Walking on the rocks instead of being on the rocks.

Richard continued to progress, and by 1998 he had reached his goal weight of 260 pounds. He had shed almost exactly half his weight. He had regained his mobility. He had resurrected his life. He had re-inflated his self-esteem. He had reinvented himself so successfully that people mistook him for his younger brother. Even Richard couldn't quite believe it.

"I was sure it would happen. I just wasn't sure I would get down to 260," he says.

At times of doubt—of which there were many—Richard had consoled himself with one thought. "If I had learned to walk again and beat those odds, then I knew I could do anything," Richard says. "I've learned that you can do anything you set your mind to."

Many of life's failures are people who did not realize how close they were to success when they gave up. – Thomas Alva Edison

Going the Extra Mile—Karen Preston

*Karen Preston's story not only shows what can be achieved once
commitment to a goal is made, but it also provides some
wonderful practical tips on how to make eating and the approach
to food a very positive experience.*

---

*Obesity runs on both sides of my family. My parents never said anything about
my weight, so I didn't really think about it when I was young. Even in those
days most people did not know about nutrition, and my parents were no exception, so we had a diet rich in cholesterol and fat. My mother was impressed with
the nutritional value of milk, and the four of us kids would drink seven gallons
of milk a week between us!*

We moved around the country a lot, and I changed schools several
times. By the time I landed in sixth grade, however, I was at a school
and an age where my weight began to bother me. Actually it wasn't so
much my weight as my overall size. I was very tall—almost always the
biggest in my class—and this created problems as I entered adolescence
and a new school.

I was enrolled in an affluent public school, and some of the other
kids, especially the boys, were really mean and nasty about my size.
They called me names like "butterball" and "truck," and it really hurt.
In retrospect, I really wasn't that overweight, but I might as well have
weighed ten tons for the treatment that I received. One of the worst
humiliations was a class weighing where we all trooped to the gym to
be weighed and had our weights publicly announced. I was humiliated.

I felt like two different people. At home, the second of four siblings,
I was outgoing, a peacemaker, and a sweet, good kid. Outside the
home, I was shy and reserved. I had a couple of friends but not much

social life.

My first attempt at weight loss, when I was in the seventh grade, was on an egg and tomato diet. I survived that for two weeks, dropping twenty pounds in the process before I quit. Of course, all of the weight came back, and I developed a taste aversion to hardboiled eggs!

One girl who had previously been very mean about my weight changed her attitude completely. It was then that I realized how much prejudice there is against overweight people.

I continued in the same community, doing well academically, but I hated being there. I disliked it so much that I worked extra hard and graduated a year early so I could escape. I never felt that I belonged. I realize now that I am a very social person that needs others to bring the best out of me.

College was a good experience for me. People were friendly and respectful, and I felt as if I belonged there. I did gain fifteen pounds during my college years, but I also met my husband, Paul. When we married, I was about two hundred pounds and a shade under six feet tall. Paul is six feet, six inches, and had been very active, but in the early part of our marriage we got into some poor habits: eating snacks late at night and not exercising. By the time I was twenty-four, my weight had crept up to about 250 pounds. I joined Diet Workshop with a friend and proceeded to lose eighty pounds. I quit before I lost all the weight when the leader kept displaying me each week as his star student. I wasn't comfortable in that role. But I got down to 170 and felt good.

My weight pretty much stayed that way until I became pregnant in my late twenties. I drank plenty of milk during this time, but I only gained twenty-two pounds during my pregnancy. When my daughter was about two-and-a-half, my life changed dramatically.

We moved to Portland, Oregon, and the move was very hard on me. I love Portland now, but when we first moved I felt very isolated. I had moved away from my family and friends. But soon I took a job and quickly got two promotions that put me in charge of a department of twelve people. I really didn't like the administrative and human resources part of the job and felt very miserable. Sometimes I worked eighty hours a week, and I would go two or three days without seeing my daughter awake. When I quit the job, I felt miserable and as if I had failed. This was unusual for me. I have always had a positive attitude and felt that I could do anything I put my mind to, so failing at this job was a real blow. I began using food as a way to stuff down my feelings.

I then spent some time as a stay-at-home mom, but there weren't other young mothers in my area, so I felt even more isolated. Before long, the bad habits crept back in, and the weight started piling on. My next job didn't help much from that point of view. I was much happier working in childcare, but I occasionally took the kids to fast-food restaurants or baked cookies, and there seemed to be a snack or a treat at every break during the day. And at the end of the day, I was so tired that I didn't have the energy to cook a meal for the family, so it was fast food three or four times a week.

As my weight increased, I chose to ignore it. I hid the scales. I busied myself with taking care of my daughter, my husband, and the kids under my care—everyone but me. I became more withdrawn. The shy, reserved person was dominant; I didn't see much of my positive, outgoing self. It was buried under a 350-pound frame.

Over the years, I had learned to cover my weight by hiding within my clothes. By August 1997, however, I had gotten to breaking point. It was hot and miserable, and I couldn't fit into the largest jeans in the store. I wore size thirty-two talls, and I kept busting out of the zipper. I bought some sweatpants from a big and tall men's shop to wear around the house, but I was too hot! I had to face the fact that I had run out of camouflage.

When I admired a friend who had lost weight, she invited me to join her Weight Watchers group. I started off great and lost thirty-three pounds, but when my friend switched to an evening job, she could not attend anymore. I found I wasn't getting the support I wanted from the other members. The paid leader was friendly enough, but I needed more from the others. I even tried to get some support going between the group members, but there wasn't much of a response, so I quit.

I mentioned my disappointment a short time later to a couple I met on a cruise. They told me about TOPS and suggested I give it a try. I had some trepidation when I went to my first meeting, but I was totally blown away by the response I got. Four different women gave me their phone numbers and asked me to call if I had questions, wanted to go walking, or needed support. That was enough for me; I signed up that very night.

As I got to know the group members over the next few weeks, I had no doubt that I would be successful. That was three years ago. Today I am 150 pounds lighter.

In addition to choosing the right food, managing portion sizes, and exercising, nurturing myself and staying positive has been essential. This is where my fellow group members have helped me the most. They provide me with an outlet so that I no longer have to hide my feelings. With such a caring group that can identify with my issues, I don't need to hide my feelings.

As for exercising, I have to admit that I didn't do anything until about eighteen months ago. By that time I had already lost a hundred pounds. I had a foot problem called Plantar Fasciitis, which kept me from walking for exercise. This condition is often caused by wearing high heels, having flat feet or high arches, or being overweight. My doctor suggested riding a bike or swimming, but I didn't want to ride a bike at that weight, and I didn't have convenient access to a swimming pool. When our community center pool opened, however, I was one of the first there.

I started out taking water aerobics three mornings a week. On other days, I rode the stationary bikes or used the machines in the fitness room. My foot problem got better, but it didn't go away completely. Three months after the community center opened, I had to have surgery and stay off my feet for three weeks. My doctor OK'd me to exercise for five minutes per day at first. It seemed silly to drive all the way there for just five minutes, but I knew that I needed the exercise, and *I had to start a routine, or it just wouldn't happen.* So I spent twenty minutes driving to and from the fitness center to work out for five minutes!

Within a few weeks, I was walking longer and more frequently, and that's when I made a big decision. My New Year's resolution had always been to lose weight. I knew that I would reach my goal in 2000, so now I needed something new.

I decided to walk the Portland Marathon in October.

I have always felt that it was essential to make an active decision to be positive. I try to see the good things in people and try to find the positive spin on events. I did this with my weight-loss efforts, and I know that it helped me reach my goal. I use many different tactics.

I always set a beautiful table at which to eat, and I always sit down to eat even if I am having just a snack. I make sure that the table is always set with pretty plates, placemats, and candles. Occasionally I'll buy flowers for the table, and when I eat alone, I listen to slow, restful music. I pay attention to the colors and textures of the food. I am treating myself, and I want to savor the food, not just devour it.

Terrific Tactic

Always sit down to eat.

I ask for support when I need it. About two years ago, I was having trouble resisting cravings, and I was in a long weight plateau. I sat down and wrote myself a letter about why I was overweight and why I wanted to lose weight. I made three copies of the letter, sealed them in envelopes, and gave them to three members of my TOPS group. I told them not to open the letter but to give it back to me if they saw me straying. They accepted the sealed letter with good grace and enthusiasm. I never got one back from them, but I kept the original and read it over whenever I needed a boost.

I made a list of ways to pamper myself without eating. I use this list as reference when I'm having a hard time and promise myself one of the items as a reward for reaching a goal.

Terrific Tactic

Find rewards other than food, and use them as an incentive and as a way to take care of yourself. Massages, beauty care, CDs, tickets to special events—all make good rewards.

I have kept a journal for a long time. Initially, it was a traditional journal, describing my struggles and successes. Then I tried the Oprah-style gratitude journal where each evening you list five things that you are grateful for. I have since tried a success journal in which I list everything I did on a daily basis that will help me toward my goal. This really keeps me focused and positive.

I have a crystal bowl that contains some folded slips of paper. On each piece, I have written something about myself that I really like or something that I feel I do well. For example, on one it says I am persistent and on another that I am good at scrapbooking. When I am feeling crummy, I go to the bowl and pick out different slips of paper to remind myself of my strengths and to avoid getting too self-critical.

When I hear myself thinking negatively, I tell myself, "STOP!" Then I find a more positive way to express the thought.

Interrupt negative thoughts, and find more positive ways to express them.

I am a perfectionist, but as I have come to understand, none of us is perfect. We need to learn to be kind to ourselves when we slip up.

The last technique I use is visualization. I imagine myself being successful and see myself reaching my goals in a variety of situations, like buying smaller clothes or achieving an exercise goal.

Well, you are probably wondering what happened when this ex couch potato tackled the Portland marathon. I trained hard for six months. Three weeks before the event I participated in a twenty-one mile walk. My feet hurt so badly I had to practically crawl the last mile!

The marathon itself started ominously. Right at the start, the heavens opened, and it absolutely poured. My walking companion was having problems, and I had to leave her behind after the first couple of miles. Undaunted, I carried on, chatting to others and giving my support to whomever needed it.

At the three-mile mark, I came across my colleagues in the flute choir. I have been a member of the Rose City Flute Choir for one-and-a-half years, and when we were asked to perform along the route, they agreed to do it to support me. Moments before, I met two members of my TOPS group that handed off some roses I had bought the night before. When I reached my flute choir, I gave them the roses. At that moment the rain stopped.

During the fourteenth mile, I was joined by my ever-supportive husband and daughter, now fifteen. They walked with me for almost half a mile before turning back. I had a nice surprise during mile twenty-one when I was cheered on by a very good friend and TOPS member whom I respect and admire. She and her husband, who uses a wheelchair, had come out just to support me. My friend walked with me for about two blocks and then rejoined her husband.

At mile twenty-two, five members of my TOPS group were there, cheering me on. One of them was a retired nurse who offered to walk with me the last few miles. Good job she did! At mile twenty-three I hit "the wall." I felt dizzy and nauseous. Linda convinced me to eat and drink more liquid. I soon revived and experienced the exhilaration of approaching the finish line. I had done it!

My weight loss is a journey, not a destination. My purpose is not to lose weight but to get the most out of my life. I now have the freedom to do that, to do things that I never thought possible.

I am going to continue to give motivational speeches, be a preschool party entertainer, live healthy, and look after myself. Oh, and did I tell you? This summer I'm entering a triathlon.

I have not failed. I have just found 10,000 ways that don't work.
– Thomas Alva Edison

The Daily Gift of Health—Joan Lambert

Joan Lambert describes how keeping focused on the benefits and purpose of her program maintains her motivation and positive attitude.

I was skinny then, and I knew it. I remember running around in a two-piece bikini, blonde hair, blue eyes —I had the world at my feet! My dad nicknamed me, "Bones." By the time I was in the sixth grade and twelve years old, it was a different feeling —I knew I had a weight problem.

We had just moved to a very small town where new kids aren't accepted easily. This was the fifth "new" school for me. One day our teacher lined us up and marched us down to get weighed by the school nurse. After we returned to our classroom, our teacher called out our names one by one, and we had to tell out loud how much we weighed so she could record it. When I said my weight, I realized mine was the highest of all kids in the class. Everyone else realized it, too, and started laughing loudly. I cried. It hurt having them make fun of me. The next year I moved on to junior high school. The kids at school never let me forget how fat, poor, and ugly I was. It was a miserable lifestyle, being tormented on a daily basis by the same people year after year.

Growing up, we didn't have much money to spend on healthy foods but instead ate a diet of high-fat, high-volume foods like mashed potatoes with hamburger gravy, fried chicken, macaroni and cheese, etc.

When I was nineteen years old, I went to the doctor for the first time. My thyroid had stopped functioning. I didn't know why, but I was told to take medicine to control it and to lose weight because I was grossly obese. Great. I went on my first diet. It consisted of eating my favorite vegetable—canned corn—three times a day. I also swam at least one hour a day. Within a few short months, I had lost eighty-two pounds and was quite proud of my accomplishment. I had done it. My diet days were over, so I went back to my old eating habits and gained back all the weight plus more. Several years later, I lost ninety pounds and in less than two years gained it all back. I tried—and failed—again. I didn't have what it took to be successful. I married an obese man who didn't care how much I weighed, so I gave up on myself and settled for being fat.

When I was twenty-eight, I planned to have a baby but didn't plan to gain seventy pounds. After my son's birth, I tipped the scale at 306 pounds. It was again time to crack down and give my best try at losing weight. I lost maybe forty pounds but, once again, didn't have a strong commitment to myself and for getting the weight off. One year later I turned twenty-nine and with it came the diagnosis of diabetes. At twenty-nine years old, how could this be? That was a disease that killed old people! How could this be happening to me? When I thought about it, I knew how it happened. It was those endless hours of eating bags and bags of chocolate or anything else I could find. There were no limits. I was eating to soothe an unhappy marriage, a lousy job, and having absolutely no self-esteem. I was a bad person and soon fell into a deep, dark depression. How could my husband love me if I couldn't even do it myself? Diabetes was my death sentence for sure.

My marriage and the rest of my life fell apart that year. My diabetes was suffering. My test results came back, time after time, with "poor control" highlighted. I graduated from oral medications right to insulin three times a day. I was so afraid I wouldn't live to see my fortieth birthday.

My divorce gave me a fresh start. I began working on my mental health and after a year, was ready to think about tackling my weight problem—again! I didn't want to do it, though—it was too hard. I was afraid to fail. I just knew it was time.

January 20, 1996. It was my birthday and my sister, Susanne, took me to a women's health fair in Portland. This is when my life changed, and the blessings started to rain down on me. On that day, I met fitness guru Richard Simmons for the very first time. Not only did he have everyone in the coliseum sing "Happy Birthday" to me, but he also then had a long talk with me in front of the crowd and told me how I was worth it and that I could simply lose the weight if I really wanted to. It was that easy. At that same health fair I found a booth manned by TOPS members. I remembered how my parents were both TOPS members, and at that point, I was ready to try anything. I called the 800 number and joined a chapter the very next week.

After making the commitment to do this NOW for me, the first step was taken. Next, I had to learn how to lose weight, the right way, and just do it. I started out by walking fifteen minutes a day, three times a week. That is all my body could stand at a time. After a week or so, I was walking longer distances more often. I was getting stronger. I was eating sensibly and drinking so much water I thought I must be "squeaky clean" inside and out! After thirty-one months, I had lost 106 pounds of my goal. I was really blown away when I was crowned Oregon State Queen for TOPS. It was like being Miss America for a year!

To this day I am still amazed and overjoyed when I look at myself in the mirror. I spent nearly my entire life looking away when I saw how fat I was in the mirror. Now I like what I see—it is the thinner person that was always inside me, desperately wanting to come out.

My self-esteem has made a miraculous change as well. I didn't grow up learning how to express love of any kind. Giving myself a daily gift of health literally taught me how to love myself. Taking the time to care about me made all the difference. I love who I am—I can even say it out loud!

**"Taking the time to care about me made
all the difference."**

Someone once told me that I would probably have to fight my weight for the rest of my life—but wasn't it easier to fight it in a size sixteen rather than in a size thirty-two? She was right. She happened to be one of those people that "wished" they could lose the weight. Her jealousy was one of the things that motivated me to lose even more weight. She told me when I got to my goal that I had something she had wanted for years but never could have. How could she not understand that if she wanted it, she could have it?

I have met several obstacles along the way, but I didn't let any of them stop me.

Getting started was hard, not to mention expensive—boneless, skinless chicken breast and other diet foods are much more expensive. I wasn't sure I could afford this lifestyle. Then it occurred to me—am I worth it? Is my health worth it? Absolutely!

Our family was used to going out to dinner with my in-laws every Friday evening to an all-you-can-eat "chuck-wagon" type restaurant. I continued to go with them with a positive attitude each time. I was determined to eat sensibly. Then the temptation began to kick in. All of my favorite foods and all I could eat. It became such a struggle to not eat all the foods I had grown up on and loved. No one else had a problem with this—just me. I felt so alone with it. After I got mad at myself for overeating, I got selfish. *I put my foot down and stood up for myself.* I did not want to continue eating at that restaurant. This was really hard for my family to understand and was the fuel for many heated conversations. They were quite angry with me, but I had to do it if I was ever going to get to my goal. *I knew and accepted that if I didn't have the strength to eat sensibly at a buffet, I had no business being there.*

If you believe you cannot cope with a high-risk situation, avoid it.

At first, I chose to do my workout after I got home from work each day. This worked for a while, especially when my workouts were only fifteen to thirty minutes in length. But when it was increased to an hour, it was a problem. I would come home from work and be met at the door by my dog, three kids, and husband, all demanding my time. We had Boy Scouts, Girl Scouts, conferences, medical appointments, and lots and lots of ways to spend my time on them, rather than on my workout. It was becoming increasingly common that there was no time for me. *I had to find a way to chisel out an hour for myself if I was ever going to get to my goal.* I was used to getting up at 5 A.M. each day and going to bed at 9 P.M. So the hour I carved out for me was at 4 A.M. each day. It was hard to pull my carcass out of bed at that ungodly hour, but hard work always pays off. I did my workout from 4 to 5 A.M. each day, and I felt great! I had so much energy and felt so good about getting my workout done each day.

The first year of losing weight was easy compared to the second and third years. I was committed to getting healthy, and there was nothing going to get in my way. Sometime during my second year I had stopped losing weight. I was fighting the same quarter pound week after week, then month after month. I continued to exercise the same, and my eating had not changed. It was heartbreaking and frustrating—why wasn't this working anymore? I would cry when I came home from a meeting and be in a real bad mood because I had a gain. There was no explanation for it. I wanted to turn to food—and sometimes I did. Then, out of the darkness, once again, I was blessed and enlightened at the same time. Richard Simmons was in town and appeared on a local television program. I was in the audience and was allowed to ask him why this was happening to me. He said to take a good look at what I was eating—to make sure the portions were what they should be. Then, take a look at my exercise program. Was I sweating? How long had I been doing the same workout? He said if it had been for a long time, I needed to change the type of exercise I was doing. That's exactly what I did. With renewed determination, I changed from walking to step aerobics. *Now, every time I hit a plateau I change my exercise.* That is what made a difference on the scale and took me straight to my goal.

Having holiday candy around is really difficult for me. Sometimes I feel like an addict that needs a chocolate fix. After all these years of resisting temptation, I think my willpower is really being tested now. I feel weaker in this area. Here is how I deal with it. *I have to make a commitment, promise, or challenge to a friend or my family members to not eat the candy.* Challenges work for me. Last Halloween my friend, Donna, and I challenged each other to not eat any of our kids' candy—if we did, we had to pay $50 to the other person. That is such a huge price to pay. Neither of us ate any of the candy.

My most effective tool was determination. If I had a gain that week or a setback, such as an overeating binge, I shrugged it off. I considered myself back on track with the very next meal. I never let it go into a daylong or weeklong binge. I believe that when you do, it can lead to being off your program for good. I do everything in my power to stay on track and not let this get the best of me.

I focused on eating low-fat, low-sugar meals *all* of the time. Chewing gum is a very effective tool in managing my weight. When I have the urge to eat, but it isn't time to eat, I pick up a piece of chewing gum instead to satisfy the urge to chew—it works.

Use sugarless chewing gum as a first response against hunger pangs or temptation.

I look at food and exercise as a daily gift to myself of health and well-being. I wish I didn't have to be so careful about what I eat and drink, but it is my cross to bear. I love how I look and feel. I don't want to change it for the world. Nothing compares to this.

Two other thoughts have helped me retain a positive attitude. When I eat, I think about what I am eating and ask myself the question: "Is this food going to get me to my goal or take me one step further from it?" I also carry around this thought from _The Choice Is Yours_: "Choosing to change is a gift you give yourself, not a deprivation you endure."

Ask yourself: "Is this food or behavior going to get me to my goal or further away from it?"

My chapter supported me with genuine caring and kindness. I couldn't have done it without them. I have never been successful at keeping off the weight, and TOPS is the ingredient that was missing all of the other times I tried to make a difference in my life.

My improved health motivates me. For the first time in my life, my diabetes control is good. My blood sugar, blood pressure, and cholesterol levels are better than my own doctor's are—he said so himself! I have made my weight management one of my highest priorities. Life means a lot to me. I have three wonderful children and Prince Charming as a husband to live for.

Failure? I never encountered it. All I ever met were temporary setbacks. – Dottie Walters

I've Changed My Mind—Elaine LaMothe

Elaine LaMothe describes what happens when you abandon fear and make a conscious decision to be positive.

In the past, before I lost nearly sixty pounds, I was defensive and negative. Many times coworkers would make comments or there would be some conflict, and I would end up in the cafeteria eating muffins that soothed my anger but not my waistline or my soul. One time, a jealous coworker was trying to sabotage my efforts. She didn't like the fact that I was getting down to her size. She approached me and started picking me apart with questions: "How much do you weigh now? What size do you wear? How much more do you want to lose?" She pushed a muffin in front of me and told me it was okay to eat — and I did. I didn't like the intimidation but couldn't deal with it effectively.

In the past, before I lost my weight, I was defensive and negative. If I was eating in a restaurant and someone questioned what I was eating, I would feel uncomfortable and eat way more than I had planned. One time I was at a restaurant celebrating my birthday, and a relative questioned what I was eating. "Is that on your diet?" he asked sarcastically. I ended up eating much more because of that comment—and my inability to deal with it.

As I lost my weight, something happened to my negative outlook. It shrank along with my fat cells. Actually, it didn't just shrink; it was transformed.

Before, I was despondent; now, I have hope. Before, my self-esteem was low; now, I believe in myself. Before, the future looked bleak; now, hope gives me the strength to keep going. I use visualization to see a successful future. I visualized what I would look like at my goal weight for many months—my results are very close to what I imagined.

Before, I dwelt on past mistakes; now, I just learn from them. Before, I rarely smiled; now, I laugh a lot of the time. Before, I was in denial; now, I am honest with myself.

I used to be the world's greatest procrastinator; now, I don't put things off. Before, if I got off track, I would stay off track. Now, I start over immediately to get back on track. Before, I had a monochrome vision; I only saw black and white. Now, I see in color with lots of shades of gray. Before, I used to obsess and worry about details and things that might never happen. Now, I just live in today. Worrying is counterproductive.

Before, I was constantly comparing myself with others; now, I do not judge them. Before, I interrupted others; now, I listen to them. Before, I was dismissive of others; now, I treat them as I would like to be treated.

Happiness is contagious. Now my mission in life is to help others by encouraging and inspiring them. I love encouraging people. I enjoy writing words of encouragement. There is power in the written word.

Recently, there was some conflict at work. I didn't head straight to the cafeteria. I didn't cringe, and I didn't binge. Instead, I found the humor in the situation and accepted that we are all different. I smiled in recognition of that fact. I didn't feel hungry at all.

*If you don't like something change it. If you can't change it,
change the way you think about it. – Anonymous*

If My Gym Teacher Could See Me Now—Bonnie Chocallo

Bonnie Chocallo's delightful story is about the unfolding of promise and a tale of re-creation. Her tale is testimony to what can happen if you have an open mind and a positive attitude.

I had already lost the first forty pounds before I started walking. I had never exercised before. I had spent a lot of time, thought, and even a few calories working out how to avoid doing anything physical. I was a pro at that, especially in my senior year at a new high school. I spent a large part of that year working out ways to avoid going anywhere near the gym.

Now it was the day of reckoning. Spring had arrived, and I could no longer use the weather as an excuse. Actually, I had reached the point of eliminating all excuses, weather or otherwise. I was committed to losing weight, and I knew that I had to move my body to continue with my progress. I put on my walking shoes and headed out the door. Not very far out of the door. Just down the road a little way and back. I made it. I was a little out of breath, but I was still alive. Not too bad, really.

My first goal was to walk to the end of the road, a distance of 2.7 miles. It might as well have been a marathon. But the idea seized my imagination, and after a few walks down the road it became my goal. "Some day," I told myself, "I'll get to the end of the road."

As I went on my walks, I started to feel not only physically better but also mentally stimulated. I felt a great sense of accomplishment that spurred me on. Before long, my fitness had improved. One day, I just kept walking and walking, and I made it to the end of the road. I had forgotten that I also had to walk back! It was my first five-mile walk. Reaching the end of the road was just the beginning for me.

A friend then suggested that together we enter a charity walk to raise funds for diabetes treatment. The walk was around a nearby lake, and I liked the idea of walking and raising money for a good cause. We entered the race and walked for others less fortunate than ourselves. My friend hated it and quit half way through. I loved it.

While walking in this event, raising money for charity, something wonderful happened to me. I met a delightful man named Earl McCarty. Earl was in his seventies but incredibly fit, an elegant man who was a retired bank president. As we were walking, he engaged me in conversation.

"Do you know that you have a very steady stride?" he said.

I honestly hadn't thought about *how* I walked; I had just been focusing on actually getting out there and doing it. Earl proceeded to tell me about the local race-walkers club. I knew nothing about race-walking, let alone that my area was a hotbed of activity with many regional, national, and even international events staged right in my own backyard.

Once I joined the race-walking club, I met many new friends. I liked the competition even though that was a part of me that had rarely been noticeable. Perhaps that was to do with my increased level of self-esteem. The accomplishment of doing the physical exercise was a huge incentive and reward.

By this time, I was walking at 6:30 every morning regardless of the weather. I walk in snow, ice, sub-zero temperatures—the weather has become irrelevant as has the "whether." Whether I will walk is no longer a question. I particularly like facing new physical challenges and feeling the improvement with practice. For example, there is one very steep hill near my house, and the first time I walked up it, I became very fatigued and light-headed. But within a few days, I was walking up that hill without problems.

What I like about walking is that it's free and it is a natural activity. I encourage people to start with baby steps and feel the accomplishment of getting stronger, fitter, and faster. If you take this sensible approach, there's no reason to get hurt. I have never had a serious injury.

I have placed well in a number of prestigious events. In an international event, I came in second in my age group. I was on such a high that when I left to drive home, I headed the wrong way and had to take a detour of eight miles to get home!

All of my walking helped me lose another forty-two pounds, a loss of eighty-two pounds in all. If I would not walk, I know that my weight would balloon again. The walking has also given me confidence and strength that I did not know I had.

My walking has taught me that there are no excuses. In one race, I somehow got a stone in my shoe, and it was rubbing against my heel and causing discomfort. I was trying to ignore it, and I certainly wasn't going to stop and lose valuable position and time that would be impossible to make up. As I rounded one corner, Earl was there to cheer me on.

"Looking good," he yelled as I tried to keep pace with the leading group.

From that point on I can honestly say I forgot the stone and the discomfort. I blocked it out, increased my pace, and won the race.

I have come to realize that many things in life are like that stone in the shoe. You can use the discomfort as an excuse to quit, or just carry on toward the finishing line the best you can. If you keep going, sometimes you will win, and you will always feel good about yourself.

Whether you think you can or think you can't, you're right.
– Henry Ford

Rankin's Reminders

Accentuate the Positive

Have hope. Your potential is limitless. Reach out, and grab it.

Learn from other people's mistakes. There's not enough time for you to make them all.

Look on the bright side. Find the positive aspects in every event. You never really know what an event means at the time it's happening, so make a decision to turn it into a positive.

Don't worry. Worrying achieves little. It is negative energy spent on things that may never happen.

See the humor. Try to find the funny side. You cannot be miserable while you are laughing.

Don't procrastinate. Carpe diem—"Seize the day!"

Face fears. If you can have the courage to face your worst fears, you won't be forever running from them and thus controlled by them.

Chapter 4

Weight and the Mind-Body Connection

Understand how the unconscious can control eating

*The body is the actual outward manifestation, in physical space,
of the mind. – Candace Pert*

Nearly fifteen years ago, I met a client who was to have a profound influence on my practice and my thinking about human nature. I was clinical director of the weight-loss program at that time, and as such was immersed in behavior-modification techniques and lifestyle change issues. The specific role of the subconscious in behavior hardly crossed my mind — at least my conscious mind. I was concerned with more practical issues. Until Jan entered my office.

She was unbelievably anxious the first time we met and hardly spoke. Painfully and slowly, the horrific details of her current and former life emerged. As the details of unthinkable sexual, physical, and emotional abuse from virtually every major figure in her life emerged, Jan would fade in and out of consciousness, sometimes passing out, sometimes seemingly stuck in a catatonic state.

I had my notions about what was happening but soon called my trusted colleagues for consultation. I contacted the University of Pennsylvania Hospital, which I knew to be the best program in the country for these types of problems, and got supervision. I read books and journals and attended seminars on the subject. My diagnosis was confirmed. Jan had multiple personality disorder.

It took almost ten years for us to unravel the complex of more than fifty alter egos that had kept Jan sane for more than forty years. There were confused, terrified, and broken child alters; out-of-control adolescents who wanted to cut themselves; mature teenagers who could take control; raging and suicidal personalities; seductive girls; loving, caring women; and even two males.

In this disorder, each alter ego is the guardian of a secret, a secret so horrific that the conscious mind cannot deal with it. Trapped in the unconscious, this ego state has incredible emotional energy and occasionally, when appropriately triggered, tries to force itself into consciousness. There then ensues a tremendous battle as the subconscious tries to force its way up into awareness and the conscious tries to keep it down in the dark recesses of the mind. The battle creates tremendous anxiety, flashbacks, panic attacks, depression, and other dissociative phenomena, like out-of-body experiences and amnesia.

The ideal way to treat this problem is to take each alter and bring its secret into consciousness, thus defusing its emotional power. When an alter is thus defused, there is no need for the amnesic barriers that were set up to maintain her secret, and the alter can be integrated into the system. If this process continues, the theory goes, eventually the whole system can be integrated, thus completely eliminating the psychiatric symptoms that characterized the condition. Complete integration is not the only legitimate goal of therapy. Having the client get control of the system, and leading her life as the chairperson of the board of the alter group, is also a legitimate therapeutic goal.

The process of defusing an alter, of bringing its horrendous secret into consciousness against the most tremendous resistance, is like taking days to deliver a baby who could explode at any moment. The memories and emotions are raw, primitive, and potentially lethal. They are the experiences of a child, exactly as they were experienced at the time of the trauma. Each alter also has her own physical characteristics—specific handwriting, appearance, and physical symptoms. If Jan came to my office complaining of a migraine, I knew which alter was around, and by using hypnosis, I could defuse the situation. One alter suffered from stomach pains, another from leg cramps, and so on. Alters also have different voices that often reverberate around consciousness in a very loud voice, demanding attention. Often there are furious fights among the alters. Much of the time the person can hear these voices and participate in the discussion, what is called co-consciousness. Those of us who do not have a dissociative disorder have much fainter voices, almost echoes, and we call them intuition.

Alters don't just have physical characteristics and symptoms; they have behavioral ones, too. Some binge wildly; others are almost anorexic. Some don't care about food; others are obsessed about it. If you ever had doubts about the notion that the subconscious is reflected in the body, they would be quickly dispelled if you were to observe therapeutic work with a multiple personality.

Jan and I were on this voyage for more than ten years. Gradually we defused the alters, getting them to give up their horrific secrets. Gradually we worked farther and farther down the system, peeling back the layers of fear, and getting to the core, and worst, experiences. For me, this whole therapeutic process was humbling, revealing, and rewarding. A decade after we started, Jan was integrated.

What does all this have to do with weight control? A lot, in my view.

First, you need to know that the term Multiple Personality Disorder has been replaced with the term Dissociative Identity Disorder (DID). This recognizes the fact that the problem is not the *existence* of different ego states or alters but the *fragmentation* of the system. All of us have different ego-states—we can be moody, playful, energetic, etc. Most of us have a sense of integration—we are conscious of these states and seem to move relatively freely between them. We are integrated, not fragmented. *What Jan and others suffering from DID show so dramatically is the impact that our ego-states have on our behavior.*

If you visit a dissociative disorders inpatient unit, you will find that about 90 percent of the patients are obese and that the other 10 percent are anorexic. The relationship between early childhood trauma (especially sexual and physical abuse) and eating disorders has been well documented.

A child's coping is limited and comforting herself with food is one of the few available options. Eating and food are a good distraction to intrusive traumatic thoughts and memories. Excessive weight is a barrier to intimacy. Shame, guilt, and disgust are characteristic feelings of the abused that not only drive excessive eating but also lead to a horrific self-image that finds expression as severe obesity. Moreover, there is an ego state inside every severely abused child that hates her body because it was violated and because it let her down. What better way is there to punish it than by crushing it with extra weight?

In an organization of a quarter million members dedicated to helping people lose weight, there will be many members who were abused as children, and a few of these will have a Dissociative Identity Disorder. Dawn Counts is one of them. In her story, you will see that she has learned to control those ego-states that threaten her program, either by binging or other forms of sabotage. Because of the nature of her condition, Dawn can easily identify which part of her mind is creating the problem. Years of fragmentation enable her to isolate and identify the cause of behavior. If you don't have a dissociative disorder, then the task of identification and control is more difficult. Finding out which part of you is destructive to health is a critical part of the success puzzle. If you can't identify it and learn to control it, then it will control you.

Some emotional eating falls into the category of dissociative eating and prompts the question, "Who is doing the eating?" A woman is dedicated and committed to her program and then gets angry. Before she knows it, she is eating out of control—stuffing the emotion down by inhaling hundreds of calories she doesn't even taste. This is not the rational behavior of an intelligent woman committed to a program of health and sensible eating—someone else is doing the eating. She needs to address that part of her, whether it is the frightened child or the churning adolescent, and take adult control. Unless she finds a more mature way to handle the anger, this self-destructive "coping" strategy will prevent her from ever reaching her goals.

One fascinating dimension of these ego states is how the control of them can improve health. We know that the mind and body are an interconnected system and that the mind and body communicate with each other at several levels. There is an incredibly complex network that allows for the sharing of information at a molecular level, which prompted Candace Pert, a pioneer of mind-body medicine, to write:

> *In the popular lexicon, these kinds of connections between body and brain have long been referred to as "the power of the mind over the body." But, in the light of my research, that phrase does not accurately describe what is happening. Mind doesn't dominate body, it becomes body—body and mind are one. I see the process of communication that we have demonstrated, the flow of information throughout the whole organism, as evidence that the body is the actual outward manifestation, in physical space, of the mind. ... And when we explore the role that emotions play in the body, as expressed through the neuropeptide molecules, it will become clear how emotions can be seen as a key to the understanding of disease*
> *(Molecules of Emotion, p.187).*

When you get angry, a cascade of chemicals flow through the body, influencing many physical processes. If anger is suppressed, this cascade is likely to last longer and have a more chronic effect throughout the body. This in turn will affect the immune system, increasing vulnerability at various points of the body and raising the risk of diseases like cancer and heart disease. Managing that raging child inside not only has the behavioral benefits that come from less binging, healthier eating, and better exercise, but it also has physical benefits derived from a calmer, more balanced mind-body.

Ego states not only can come and go on a moment-to-moment basis. You can be stuck in the rut of one for many years. Thought and behavior can be so habitual that it can be difficult ever to achieve enough forward momentum to shed that particular skin.

Shedding a negative identity can create enormously positive forces that affect the mind-body. Being exposed to the right environment at the right time can bring dramatic changes. Social environments create identities, helping us to make the connection, physically and psychologically.

Identities are formed in the most important social environment, the family. The roles that we adapt in our family as a child become our characteristic ways of dealing with the outside world. In the right social environments, ones that inspire trust and safety, dormant potential can come to life.

It does take something special to achieve escape velocity and leave behind the destructive legacies of childhood experiences and identities. It is often a lifelong battle but one that has to be fought if you are going to succeed. Controlling the darker, negative sides of the self and marshaling positive energy has tremendous consequences for mind, body, and spirit.

Reading Lessons—Cindy Callis

Cindy Callis, a quite remarkable person, experienced an amazing transformation when she found herself in a group of people that brought the best out of her. Did her ability to socialize, read, and take control of her life suddenly develop, or was it there all the time, lurking in her mind-body just waiting to be switched on?

Cindy Callis is the fourth of six children. Cindy is not like any of her four brothers or her sister. She never was. As a baby it literally took her forever to be able to hold her head up. Some forty years later she can, metaphorically and physically, very definitely hold her head up.

Although she was somewhat delayed in her developmental milestones, with the help of her loving siblings—who used to hold her up for support—Cindy was able to learn to walk and talk. Her parents knew, however, it was going to be a long haul. They hoped it would. The doctors weren't sure the haul was going to be that long. They didn't expect Cindy to live past the age of fifteen.

Cindy was born with Down's syndrome. Her childhood was difficult. She suffered from seizures and had hypoglycemia but never seriously enough that hospitalization was required. She went to a special education class but was very isolated and had no friends. By the time she was an adolescent she had gained weight. She became more and more isolated. She talked little, didn't read, and hardly ever went out.

This trend continued into her thirties. Living at home with mom, Dean, and dad, Charles, Cindy became a recluse. A heavy recluse. She was five feet, two inches tall, and weighed nearly 250 pounds. She couldn't move around very easily and could barely lie down in comfort. About all she did was stay at home, watch television, and gain weight.

Cindy was very close to Charles, who was retired by now. But it was when Dean had a heart attack that Cindy started to be concerned about her own weight. Following her heart attack, Dean changed her eating habits and lost twenty-five pounds on her own before joining TOPS. Dean's sister had joined TOPS, and now she and Cindy started attending. The idea of joining a group of strangers terrified Cindy. The idea of talking about her weight was a daunting prospect. The idea of talking at all was completely alien.

No doctors had suggested that Cindy lose weight. But she was self-conscious about her weight. One time, she broke the front seat of her parent's van and from that day will never sit in the front seat, although, of course, it has long since been repaired!

At Cindy's first meeting she sat with her head down, making no eye contact whatsoever. Not that her behavior discouraged the members of the group from encouraging her. They hugged her, talked with her, and included her. Slowly, week by week, Cindy came out of her shell. And some of the shell dropped away. She lost seven pounds the first week.

The TOPS meetings became the focus of Cindy's life. It seemed like for the first time in her life she had found a purpose.

As she said, "I'm different there."

Soon Cindy—the woman who never had a friend, who could barely communicate—was interacting with the other TOPS members. She loved the people at the meeting, which explains why her mother would drive nearly a hundred miles every Tuesday night so that she could attend the meeting.

Embarking on her weight crusade, some remarkable things started to happen to Cindy. Having never eaten fruits and vegetables in her life, she started eating carrots and pears. Previously silent and noncommunicative, Cindy couldn't be kept quiet at meetings. More remarkably, Cindy, who had never read before, began to read nutrition labels. Not only read them but also understand them and apply the information appropriately.

**Don't just read nutrition information; apply
it to your situation.**

As Dean says about Cindy, "Her life began when she joined TOPS."

Once in the program, Dean began preparing healthy meals, and Cindy began to exercise. She started walking and before long was on a treadmill three times a day for thirty minutes at a time.

By the end of the first year, Cindy had lost eighty-six pounds.

She was the runner-up queen for the state of Kentucky. This meant that the formerly reclusive Cindy had to go on stage in front of hundreds of people. She handled it like a pro. In fact, she was such a hit that no one wanted her to leave the stage. Her mom lost count of the standing ovations.

The same thing happened the following year. By now, Cindy was not only losing weight, but she was also getting fitter and more active. Previously completely dependent on her mom, Cindy started to prepare not just her food but food for her parents, too.

When Cindy's dad had a heart attack, she was in much better shape to help. Whereas previously Cindy had to be taken care of, now she was becoming the caretaker.

Cindy now looks after both ailing parents. She does everything around the house—laundry, dishes, meals, etc., and even makes sure that her parents have taken their medications! And she also ensures that every Tuesday night she drives the hundred-mile round trip to the TOPS meeting. The girl whom doctors said wouldn't live past fifteen is now taking care of her parents.

*People often say that this or that person has not yet found
himself. But the self is not something one finds, it is something
one creates. – Thomas Szasz*

A Song for All Seasons—Rhoddie Ludwig

Rhoddie Ludwig tells the story of a child who could either be creative, confident, and musically talented or one with no self-esteem, crushed by weight. The transformation of her identity from the negative, unfulfilled one into the positive, creative one is a testimony to both how identity can be changed and how long it can take.

Rhoddie Ludwig was an overweight child. Raised in Vermont she was the apple of her father's eye. In her happy childhood, her weight did not bother her too much. Her father did not have a weight problem; neither did her sister, of whom Rhoddie was somewhat envious. Sister was mom's favorite. Mom herself was just four feet, eleven inches tall, and was slim. Dad loved music and had a wonderful voice. And so did Rhoddie.

By the time she was fourteen, the family had relocated to Florida. By this time Rhoddie had grown unhappy with her weight, unhappy with being chosen last for sports, and unhappy with a lack of male attention. But she had grabbed the attention of one man. The band director recognized a talent when he heard one and encouraged Rhoddie to sing. Before long he was secretly getting her gigs at local clubs.

Rhoddie loved singing. As she puts it, "Singing compensated for my weight."

Singing did more than that. It allowed her to express herself and show people what lay beyond her weight. As her singing "career" started to take shape, so did Rhoddie. In the summer of her junior year she lost seventy pounds.

In the fall, her outside activities were keeping her busy and happy. She now even had a stage name, "Misty Warren," partly required to hide the real fact of her identity and age. Fifteen-year-olds weren't meant or allowed to be singing in nightclubs.

Her gigs meant some late nights, as well as lost sleep for her and her band director-mentor. Rhoddie was sometimes a little bleary-eyed in school, but for her mentor the cost was much higher. Driving home late one night, he fell asleep at the wheel, drove into a quarry, and died instantly.

Rhoddie was devastated. The gigs stopped. She had a hard time singing—even in the shower. Within four months, she gained forty pounds. Before long singing had stopped altogether, and Rhoddie went back to being a regular teenager. A regular, fat, teenager.

Upon graduation from high school, Rhoddie had lost her direction. Lacking enthusiasm for anything else, she followed her sister's footsteps and joined the Navy. Or tried to. After discovering that she was too heavy to be accepted, she lost sixty pounds in six months on a steady diet of diet pills.

Once accepted into the Navy, she was stationed in San Diego. There she met her husband and before long she was busy quickly raising a family. Very quickly. Two children in eighteen months. She gained sixty pounds while pregnant and became addicted to diet pills prescribed while she was pregnant. When taken off these pills, she experienced severe withdrawal symptoms that lasted several weeks.

Needless to say, singing and entertaining were taking a back seat to bottles, diapers, and play dates. And the weight continued to rise alarmingly.

Her weight had increased to over three hundred pounds, but her height had stayed the same, five feet, two inches. Rhoddie didn't notice, or if she did, she decided not to pay attention. Rather she turned her attention to a medical career upon receiving her degree, an occupation that could be portable because of her husband's military career.

Using the GI bill to good effect, she went to college when her children were still at a preschool age and pursued a career in medical administration. Over the next few years, she graduated and began her career. Soon she was compulsively diving into her work, adding it to her other addiction. She continued to be a sneak eater, denying her weight and eating "even though I was not hungry."

To this point Rhoddie had not even thought about her weight. And then one day there was one of those pivotal motivating moments that threatens to change your life. It was the first of three that Rhoddie would have.

Rhoddie was proud of her work and dressed the part. One day one of the patients at the clinic where she worked remarked in all sincerity, "You dress very nicely for a fat lady."

Something clicked. A fat lady. Rhoddie looked in the mirror and didn't like what she saw. For the first time since high school, she was motivated to try to lose the weight. Not just motivated, but also desperate. It's almost as if she had been holding back the floodwaters of her motivation, and now they burst through the dam.

She then embarked on a search for the Holy Grail. Pills hadn't been the answer. Now Rhoddie went on a staple diet—two of them, in fact.

One person, a psychiatrist, suggested the technique of inserting a staple in her ear. The theory was that thirty minutes before eating, wiggling the staple back and forth for five minutes would deter any "need" for food—presumably some weird offshoot of acupuncture. It didn't work.

Rhoddie also seriously considered having a jejunum bypass, a procedure in which the major portion of the large intestine is removed. This was being offered widely in San Diego at this time, and Rhoddie was enthusiastic to do it. Fortunately for her, CHAMPUS, the medical insurance organization, wasn't enthusiastic at all. Personally knowing Jean Stacy, whose story appears on page 155, Rhoddie now says, "Thankfully I didn't go through with it."

As the Holy Grail failed to materialize, so did Rhoddie's weight loss. Soon she slipped back into denial until two incidents revived her motivation by bringing her face to face with stark reality.

She and her husband took their two children and their friends to

Magic Mountain, an amusement park near Los Angeles. It was the first week it had reopened since an unfortunate accident had claimed the life of a rather obese woman aboard "The Colossus," a large roller coaster. Three months earlier, an obese woman, intoxicated at the time, had released the safety belt and stood up when the Colossus was at one of the peaks of the ride, and she was thrown to her death. Being among the first to arrive at the park, Rhoddie's party immediately headed for the Colossus. As they started to board one of the attendants walked over to Rhoddie and, quite embarrassed, asked her to "take a test." Posted over the coaster car was a sign stating that if you were pregnant, had heart problems, or were overweight you must take a test. The test consisted of securing a safety belt and pulling a bar across your lap. Rhoddie passed the bar and failed the belt.

She was told she could not ride the Colossus. She told her family and friends to go ahead on the ride. As she walked away, she noticed a television crew headed her way. A reporter asked if she minded being interviewed.

"Always the entertainer, I said, no, of course not," says Rhoddie.

They asked if she felt she was discriminated against because she was not allowed on the ride. She said that she realized and accepted that it was a safety precaution.

"It's not their fault I'm overweight. I'll just have to lose the weight and come back," she said right into the camera.

Immediately afterward some of the management team at the park approached her and praised her positive interview. She's never been back.

The interview aired that evening on Los Angeles TV station KNBC, which reaches San Diego. Her phone rang off the hook with calls from friends who had viewed it. None asking how she felt, only about the comedy that she interjected during the interview.

The interview and the embarrassment were felt and, deep down, perhaps without knowing it, led to the next happening. A short time later a third motivating moment occurred, which really did change

Rhoddie's life. It was close to September and football season.

Rhoddie is a big football fan, and it was her Sunday tradition in the fall to relax in her favorite chair and watch the Chargers.

"As the lineup was being announced the defensive linemen were introduced along with their photos and weights. I realized that I WEIGHED MORE THAN MOST OF THEM!! Why it never set in before is a wonder.

"As I sat up in my chair that fateful Sunday afternoon, staring at the screen, looking at the numbers beside each of the players' names, I started to cry. Not outwardly, but inside.

"You see, I truly never admitted that I really weighed in excess of three hundred pounds. For some reason, the reality of that weight I buried deep inside while outwardly I appeared a happy individual, content in my job, my family and, I thought, myself."

Touchdown!

Here she weighed more than a defensive lineman and, as she puts it, "she wasn't even in uniform." Of course, she was in a uniform of sorts, but it was a very heavy one that was pulling her down.

So Rhoddie was in a more receptive and less self-deceptive frame of mind when she saw an advertisement for a local TOPS chapter. She decided to give it a try. After all, she had tried everything else, and nothing had helped her. She was frustrated that THESE ATTEMPTS didn't work—not realizing that it was she who had to MAKE them work.

Rhoddie was impressed by the welcome she received at TOPS. She felt that the other members really understood her, but she didn't exactly feel as if she belonged. She was the heaviest person there, and after a few weeks she stopped going.

It would be another six months before Rhoddie would try again. Yet back she went, and this time she stayed—thanks to the constant phone calls of the new friends she had made in her group.

The major difference is that she stayed long enough to make friendships and to feel a sense of belonging to the group. Ricki Gibson—herself a successful member who had lost 120 pounds and had been the area queen—became Rhoddie's mentor. She would call Rhoddie every week to ensure that she was staying on track.

"Her achievement made ME want to do the same. I had the same amount to lose as Ricki had," says Rhoddie.

Find a role model who has lost an amount of weight similar to what you want to lose.

Gradually the weight started to roll off. Rhoddie lost ninety pounds in six months. Finally after all those years of sticking to a "diet," exercising—slowly at first, then graduating to walking four miles a day—really made the difference.

Rhoddie would walk the high school track in the evening so that no one would see her in shorts. There was that fat person who was still embarrassed by her appearance.

Once the weight came off, Rhoddie's voice came back. Encouraged by her TOPS pals, she started singing again—slowly at first but gradually stronger and stronger. More and more gigs throughout the Southwest.

As Rhoddie says, "I wasn't ashamed to be on stage any longer."

Rhoddie's confidence returned. So much so that she entered an audition for *Catch a Rising Star*. She thought auditions were a thing of the past for her, but she HAD to do this one. *Catch a Rising Star*, nationwide, was for YOUTH. However, this year they had opened it to "the mature" category. After making the first audition, then the semifinals, and finally the finals, she won the Mature Category!!!

"The recognition from the members was such a boost to my ego. I am now proud to say that I am a board member of La Jolla Stage

Company, producers of *Catch A Rising Star* in the San Diego area, and every year Stage Director and entertainer during each *Catch A Rising Star* performance."

Not that keeping the weight off was easy. Like so many, Rhoddie could never quite get down to her goal weight, never get rid of the last eight pounds. She stuck with it though, keeping up her walking and going to every meeting.

It was the friendship and overwhelming support that kept Rhoddie on track this time—that and the singing. As long as Rhoddie was singing, she was the person she wanted to be.

Finally, reaching her goal weight after twenty-four years, Rhoddie is now an inspiration for others, not just with a singing voice but also a talking one. As she travels the West giving motivational speeches, she gives her audiences three pieces of advice:

"Start liking yourself."

"Get into a program with people who can relate to you. It can be very lonely trying on your own."

"Set small attainable goals."

It took Rhoddie twenty-four years to reach her goal. What did she learn?

"That I'm one hell of a nice person," she says.

Isn't that strange? Everyone around her knew that all along. It just took her time to allow herself the confidence and freedom to be herself. She knows that keeping the weight off is always a struggle, but with increased confidence from her singing and speaking, don't bet against her. It may not be over 'til the fat lady sings, but this singing lady isn't fat any more.

It's not only the most difficult thing to know yourself, but the most inconvenient. – Josh Billings

Many Voices—Dawn Counts

Dawn Counts describes how she has been able to control her many alter egos and how that has helped her get control of her eating and her weight.

My system (forty-five total alters that I am aware of) works as a team. "We" do a lot of committee work and stay on target that way. Eating on a food plan has been a challenge to "the system" because "the littles" sometimes want "treats." We have agreed to color books and Barbie stuff instead of food treats. I do not lose time as badly as I once did. I have a lot of co-consciousness.

After a lifetime of shame-based food addiction, and playing the yo-yo syndrome up and down the scale, I found myself in a wheelchair because my weight had gotten so high that my body could no longer support it. My depression was immense, and my knees and back were aching so badly that I sought medical attention. I went to the doctor's office where they had to get me onto a scale that looked like something one would weigh cattle on. Not only did they have to use this huge, platformed scale, but also had to add a special weight to the thing to get an accurate reading of my weight, which was 429. To add insult to injury, when they tried to help me onto the examining table, I tipped it over. After this visit, I went home, locked myself in my bathroom, and proceeded to take the entire bottle of my son's antidepressants because I was so ashamed and wanted to die.

As I sat there, waiting to die, I looked around that tiny bathroom, and my mind started to go wild. They were going to have to tear out the wall to get me out of there. The humiliation that my sons would have to bear for that would be immense. It would take several strong men to get my body out of there. On and on my mind went, so I proceeded to use my old faithful bulimic tool of vomiting and "got rid" of the pills. Instead of death, I chose life.

I called my therapist, whom I hadn't seen in almost a year, and set up an appointment. She directed me to a support group for compulsive overeaters and food addicts, and by August 1, 1998, I had committed to eating a weighed and measured food plan, abstaining from sugar, and gaining a new life. My current weight is 257, and I am still working my "weigh down" the scale. I am doing it slowly and with lots of support so that I never again have to go back. For today, I am grateful for all of the support that I find out in the "real" world and that I didn't take my life in the isolation of that lonely bathroom on April 23, 1998.

Terrific Tactic

When your eating is out of control, seek professional help.

I am personally a compulsive overeater and food addict. I am absolutely an emotional eater. The worst part of this is the vicious, shame-based circle. The pattern for me was this: I felt like a failure, a bad person, not good enough for love (even self-love); therefore I ate to comfort myself. The more I ate, the larger I got. The larger I got, the more ashamed I was for looking like a fat slob, being a failure at keeping my weight down, so I ate to make myself feel better. Around and around this negative spiral went. There is also an incredible amount of anger-based eating. If I am angry at someone, I have been conditioned through past abuse not to lash out at them. Therefore, I eat to push down those feelings of anger. I ate away the rage. Then I looked in the mirror, and the rage turned inward. The more the rage, the more the eating. I also ate to build a wall of protection for myself. As a victim of sexual abuse, I secretly believe that part of me thought that if I were fat, no one would "want" me anymore. This is false.

My sexual abuse was horrific. The only way I could cope was escaping the situation. While my body was being abused, I left it. My mind floated around the room, and I could look down in a detached manner at what was happening to me. Sometimes I left the room altogether, and my mind left my body to go to happier places, like the beach and the fairground. The more this happened, the more I became more fragmented. I was aware of different voices in my head. They were all distinct and had different viewpoints.

It was no surprise when I was officially diagnosed with MPD. I had been trying to hold it all together for many years, not letting anyone in on my secret. Finally, talking about it was a relief. I learned more about my alters and how to control them and the whole system. I gradually got more control, taking charge of the alters and working on getting them all on the same page.

I have one alter, Dawn Robin, who is very much a bulimic. She likes to control everything in life. She loves exercise and would use that since "we" are not allowed to binge or purge.

I have about fifteen "littles." They do not control eating, but they are willing to work with the program and food plan that I have. In order to satisfy their needs (I have been good; therefore I deserve a treat—the mentality that they were raised with), I indulge them with occasional Barbie clothes or color books, etc.

I have several "teenagers." Herein lies my biggest struggle. Two of them are serious self-abusers. Cutting is another addiction of mine. I have been abstinent from cutting for several months and hope to remain that way. These "teenagers" are the ones that tend to want to "cheat." They want things like potato chips and pizza. We simply have to remind them that we are all working as a committee to get the body to a healthy state and that cheating is not allowed. That usually means we have to do something to distract them, like watch a horror film or go out to the movies or something "fun."

I have two male alters. Neither of them seems interested in food. I have never had any contact with one of them (a protector) and only know of him because the others and my therapist tell me about him. The other's—"Ralph Jones"—sole purpose is to protect and entertain the "littles," so he has no use of dieting or anything else.

The adult alters are various. There is the Gatekeeper, who simply keeps the system orderly, and Angel the Storyteller, who entertains the "littles." Then there are those that I really only know through others in the system. All I know is that we hold regular "committee meetings," and during these times I "go in" and "we" work on making sure that the whole system is working in compliance with the food plan and the "way of living" that we have committed to. No cutting, no abusive behaviors, no inappropriate "coming outs." I am very blessed in that we work well as a team, thanks to eight years with a wonderful therapist and the fact that I am co-present "most" of the time. There are times that I do lose time, but everyone seems to keep tabs on one another. If someone were to cheat—and it can and does happen on occasion—someone will tell on them. This system has allowed me to lose over 170 pounds and, for once in my life, I feel in control.

There is no such thing as a self-made man. We are made up of thousands of others. – George Adams

The Invisible Puppeteer—Kelly Alario

Kelly Alario describes the development of binging in great detail and offers hope by showing how she identified, and learned to control, that part of her that was desperate to get as much food as possible.

When I was much younger, my cousin and I were very close. He was short and skinny, and I was about a foot taller and chubby. No one believed that we were only three months apart. Our mothers are sisters, but for some reason, our individual families have very opposite eating habits. My aunt has always served normal portions of food in well-balanced meals. My mom sought fast-food meals or frozen dinners and allowed us to eat whatever portions we wanted if we begged hard enough. My cousin often did not want to eat and ate very little from his plate. I, however, loved to eat and made sure not a single pea or grain of rice was left.

I never really liked the eating situation over at my aunt's house because I felt so restricted in how much I could eat. Once, when I was six, I was staying over there, and my aunt prepared several hot dogs and chili. She served us each one hot dog with chili on a bun. I finished my dog before my cousin and asked for another. My aunt did not hesitate, since she was aware that I did not have a problem getting enough food in my stomach. Finally my cousin left the table and left at least half of a hot dog on his plate. I didn't understand how he could not want to finish one small hot dog. I then asked my aunt for yet another hot dog.

She asked, "Kelly, are you sure you want another one? You've had two already. You can have another, but you don't have to finish it, okay?"

She fixed me a third hot dog with chili on a bun. I ate it all, no problem. A few minutes later, as she began to clean up the kitchen and pick up the food for storage, I asked for another hot dog.

She said, "Kelly, this would be your fourth hot dog! Your uncle can't even eat that many hot dogs. How can you still be hungry?"

I told her that I really didn't know why I was still hungry and that my stomach was still growling. She reluctantly gave me my fourth hot dog, and I ate all of it.

When my mother came to pick me up that evening, my aunt told her that she couldn't believe I ate four hot dogs. My mother was not stunned or surprised, but once we got home, I did get fussed for being so greedy, especially because it was in front of other people. I don't even recall feeling sick or tired, but I do remember feeling very embarrassed.

I have another cousin of similar age, and we were close. She lived with her grandmother who cooked the most fattening but best-tasting meals. My cousin was always much heavier than me. Even as a small child, she was at least thirty pounds overweight. We both developed a horrible habit of picking at each other's plates. Even though her grandmother served us identical servings of identical meals, either she or I would scoop beans and rice from each other's plates or steal a French fry here and there. I was angry when my cousin stole my food because I wanted all that was in my plate. She got angry, too. The anger was not enough to empathize with the other person and stop the picking habit.

I'll never forget the image of the two of us when her grandmother decided to bake a cake. After she added the oil, egg, and water to the dry mix and beat it, she poured the mixture into the pan. She left the mixing bowl and mixer utensils in the sink to be washed later. My cousin and I almost fought for the items in the sink because there was still mixture left in them. We used our pudgy fingers by sharing the mixing bowl to lick clean. We licked the mixer utensils and spatula. We even began using our hands to make sure we got all sides of the bowl and missed nothing. When the mixture in the bowl began to have little left, my cousin took the entire bowl for herself to finish. I was very upset that I couldn't share it with her at the end. I always kept that image in my head because it reminds me of how desperate we had become with getting and keeping food.

My mother is a sweets fanatic. She has always been prey to sugary substances, like hard candies, jellybeans, and very sweet cake icing. She had to keep a stash of candies in her own bedroom under the bed so that I would not attack them. She tried labeling all foods that we somehow "earned" for ourselves by doing errands. One day, my mother had already made pudding, put each serving in pretty glasses, and labeled each one for each family member to try out. I ate three of the four. I knew they were for someone else and that I was depriving another person of their dessert. I had rather face the consequences of the other people saying, "Kelly, why did you eat my pudding? I really wanted to try that and was looking forward to it. How could you be so greedy?" I still don't know why I did it, but once I ate my share, I felt it just wasn't enough to fill my need for it. It couldn't have stayed a sample. It had to be a meal for me.

Most of my binging experiences came right after trying to diet. I used to either starve myself for a few weeks or really sacrifice, and then I'd eat enormous meals all day long until I couldn't eat another bite. When I would diet, I would have to give up things that I like most or else I'd eat too much of it. I was usually successful at losing ten or twenty pounds at a time in a few weeks by strict discipline from small portions of low-calorie food and intense exercise twice daily. Immediately after reaching my goal, I would hunt for the foods that I loved most and eat them all within the same few days. I thought that if I did this, I would get the craving out of my system for another few weeks so that I could maintain my weight.

I was in my first year of college and at the lowest I weighed as an adult when I had a serious binging incident. I struggled with my eight hundred calorie diet for a few weeks and walked two miles each night with my roommate to get to my lowest weight. About two weeks after I reached my goal and bought new clothes, I was invited to my best friend's wedding shower. She and I bonded in high school when we both had eating problems and took nonprescription asthma medicine to curb our appetites. As adults we still kept the same yo-yo dieting habits and understood that since her wedding was coming up soon, we both had to look good to fit our dresses. We really ate too little the week before her shower so that we could eat the shower food that her mother was cooking. Her mother cooked wonderful meals that were well known in the community, and the shower food was to be just as gourmet as her usual meals.

I attended the shower, but I was so busy helping accommodate the other guests that I did not get to try all the food that I had been starving myself for. After everyone left, I helped clean the house and was offered to take home any leftover food. There was a sizable portion of lasagna left over. I took that home, plus other side dishes. I took another dish for my mother. Before going to my mother's house, I stopped at my boyfriend's house to get something, and I stayed much longer than anticipated. When I got back to the car, I realized I forgot about the food, which I smelled when opening the door. It smelled like all the flavors from the house where the shower was thrown, sort of like it was heated and ready to be eaten. I thought it may have smelled a bit stronger in my car, but I knew that I really didn't have a chance to get close to the food at the shower. I finally went to my mother's house and dropped off her plate of leftovers.

She said, "Oh, this is what I've been waiting for all day long." Her nose crinkled a few times, and she told me, "Something smells bad in here. It can't be that people ate this over there, right? I think it's the lasagna."

She told me was throwing it away after I told her I had left it in the car all day. I felt bad for not coming through with what she longed for all day.

When I got home, I was determined to eat the food anyway. I never doubted that I would eat it, even if it did smell spoiled. I denied that it was spoiled in every way possible in my mind. I convinced myself that I really hadn't stayed by my boyfriend's house that long and that the food was just cooking more in my hot car. Wouldn't that make it still safe?

I ate the whole plate of lasagna, and then I ate the side dishes and desserts plate, too. I had looked forward to enjoying those dishes for so long that nothing was going to stop me. I could not go back to my friend's house to ask for more since there was no more food left. I didn't tell anyone I ate the food until I started to feel sick. I felt very full after only eating half of the lasagna plate but kept on eating anyway. After I finished both plates, I had to lie down. At this point, the spoilage hadn't kicked in yet, but the amount of food that I had eaten was making it hard to breathe. I had to concentrate on breathing deep and allowing that feeling to subside. Then came the stomach cramps, frequent severe stomach cramps that lasted for several hours. I was nauseous for a long time. I called my boyfriend to tell him how I felt, but I couldn't say what I had done. I then called my mother, and I told her what I did because I was truly scared. She told me how foolish I was for eating the food and that I needed to consider the emergency room if the pain didn't cease. After a few hours of constant pain and worry, I began feeling better and decided not to go the hospital. How could I tell another soul that I had eaten spoiled food and so much of it? I still feel disgusted with myself today for that incident. I knew I had a serious eating problem.

Other binging incidents were not as serious, yet they brought on the same physical and emotional problems that the previous incident brought. I went to a Catholic school, and the head nun would punish the students in the cafeteria if all their food was not eaten from the plate. Of course, I had no problem finishing every plate I took, but the ideology to conserve food and not waste was embedded in my brain since then. My family never threw away food, either. I can remember attaching pseudo-personalities to food so that I would feel sorry for it and not have to throw it. Allowing myself to throw away food today is still hard to do. I have even thrown away a box of cookies in the garbage in an attempt to get it out of sight so as to not be eaten, and then I'd be digging the box up again to eat it anyway. *I felt like some other spirit took over me to perform an act so disgusting as to dig in a garbage for food when not even truly starving.* Everything I would tell myself in my head was counteracted with another carefree, "Oh, what the heck. It's only a few cookies. They're all still in the box. I'll start dieting again tomorrow. How could I throw food when people in my own town are going hungry? I paid a lot for that box of cookies."

"Oh, what the heck. It's only a few cookies. They're all still in the box. I'll start dieting again tomorrow. How could I throw food when people in my own town are going hungry? I paid a lot for that box of cookies."

My binging rages would consist of eating as much of my favorite foods as I could as quickly as possible. I would usually plan it because I knew that if I was going to eat "bad" then I wanted to eat the foods I craved most. My favorite food is pizza, then corn, burgers, and chocolate chip cookie dough ice cream. I always planned to stop at three of my favorite fast-food restaurants and get combo meals on my way home from college, which was just a two-and-a-half-hour drive, just so I could ensure I had each one. My plan was always to stop after I had eaten my favorites. I still felt sane at this point in the cycle.

I felt in control up until half of the meal would be gone. Then a sad and worried voice took over that said, "You've almost finished your meal. What are you going to eat right after this? What else is in the house?" After eating everything I had planned, I felt that I had to continue. I started on foods that I don't crave, such as sliced bread, a can of peas, boiled plain noodles, etc. I ate these foods while still feeling full from my favorites. I had no control of my eyes to search for food and hands to dig for food while I tuned out everything else around me. I ate quickly, like a squirrel chews acorns. I still couldn't pinpoint what part of me was taking over, but I know it was not my intellectual side.

I tried every way possible to talk myself out of eating, such as walking away from the kitchen or watching television.

Now, I have found better ways to control this invisible puppeteer that puts new thoughts in my head of where to look for more food. For a long time, I'd feel empty inside even while full, but my tongue, throat, and stomach ached for more, more, more. My binging could be for one hour or one day or more. I always binged in private, when no one was there to stop me, judge me, or watch me, and I always felt guilty afterward. Another voice always followed a binge that chastised me for being such a loser, freak, and pig. That's why I can't keep my favorite items in the house regularly because I know I'd go crazy. I have the potential to weigh 400 pounds plus.

T e r r i f i c   T a c t i c

Don't keep very tempting foods in the house or anywhere they are easily available.

I have more insight into why I binge now. One of my careers was being a crisis counselor for victims of domestic violence and sexual assault. I learned a great deal from that job, because although my own personal assault experiences would not classify me as a moderate or even severe victim of sexual assault, I can relate to these victims just as well.

My supervisor stressed the importance of CONTROL in the lives of victims. She explained to me that victims of assault were traumatized by an event that made them feel utterly at a loss of control and power in their lives. Control doesn't bounce back after the trauma of the attack because the fear of loss of control again never goes away. The loss of control must be dealt with in order for a victim to survive an attack and survive life without suicide. Every person has her own way to cope and empower herself. Being in control of the pain that is inflicted on oneself, deciding how much substance to put into one's body, or controlling what foods will be eaten for comfort are convenient ways to cope with the trauma and to gain control. However, victims who are abusing substances or food and who inflict pain to themselves are actually *out of control with these coping mechanisms*. The mechanisms usually start off as helpful but gradually get out of control as the methods help ease the pain of the trauma.

I believe that I overeat because I feel that food won't be there for me tomorrow. My thought is that I "have to eat it now because I might starve tomorrow." I know that the feeling that I have to fend for myself and ensure that I'm not hungry is to avoid pain. I know that my problem is ALL psychological and not physical. I know what to eat and how much to eat. I'm just afraid to do it. *I'm afraid to be hungry so I overeat to control the fear, but in turn I am OUT OF CONTROL in my eating.*

Armed with this insight and distraught at having reached 230 pounds, I finally decided to do something about my problem. I began by setting small goals, such as losing five pounds in November or ten pounds by Christmas. Before I knew it, I'd lost ten, twenty, thirty, forty, fifty, then sixty pounds, and I never felt that I was really sacrificing! The key for me was consistency and lifestyle change. I still eat the foods I love, but not as often and not as much. I practice portion control. I don't even count calories anymore because I know how much to serve myself now.

Cajuns love to overfeed themselves, and grandmothers love to cook food for you. My grandmother would cook very fattening meals for me to express her love, but I'd have to explain to her that if she wanted me to be happy, she'd have to stop cooking meals like that for me all the time. I suggested other things she could do for me instead, like buy lots of gum for Easter instead of chocolate, and it worked! I've never regretted making a decision about sacrificing a little food sometimes, but I've ALWAYS regretted making a wrong decision!

The hardest parts of setting a goal to lose are the fear of failure and the fear of forfeiting my favorite foods. The fear of failure left quickly, after only a few weeks of losing about ten pounds. The fear of giving up my favorite foods left after a few months and I had lost forty pounds, since I realized I could still live by eating less favorites less often. I eat these in safe situations where the access to those foods is limited and I don't have them available after I have eaten. *The combination of knowing I could eat my favorite foods in moderation and getting control of that sad, frightened little girl was the key to my breaking the binging habit.*

Terrific Tactic

Recognize that you can eat favorite foods in moderation, in safe situations.

I had only a few minor setbacks along the way, such as career changes, holidays, and minor sicknesses that could prevent me from eating healthy and exercising. I have had minor back surgery on a slipped disc, so cold fronts always stiffen my back and prevent me from exercising for a few days. Sometimes, the back pain is discouraging because I actually enjoy exercising now and miss it when I can't do it. There were also a few times throughout the months that I could not lose any more weight and I'd plateau in the weight loss. Soon, the weight would drop again because I never gave up. Now, I feel like I'm consistent and that I'm leading up to a goal.

I could not have made any of this progress without the incredible friendship and support from my group. Their support gave me hope and the accountability I needed to get started and stay on track during the first few months. Now, I feel as if I have broken those binging

Run with Endurance the Race Set Before You—Fran Drozdz

Fran Drozdz's story is an inspirational message about the power of belief and purpose. In the pursuit of any worthwhile purpose, belief is essential.

For the first thirty-six years of her life, Fran Drozdz had no interest in fitness. She was overweight enough to earn the nickname, "Thunder Thighs," but not obese. In early adulthood, she had her hands full with a family and constant moves. As the wife of an experienced air force pilot, she endured seventeen moves in twenty-one years, and she was frequently alone, parenting her daughter, Amy.

In her mid-thirties, while stationed in Okinawa, she decide to start running to get fit and lose the extra thirty pounds she had been carrying most of her adult life. Shortly afterward, husband Stan was relocated to Hawaii, where there are more runners per capita than anywhere else in the world. Soon after arriving in Hawaii, Fran was sitting outside, smoking a cigarette, when members of the Hickam (Air Force base) running club passed her on their monthly fun run. Fran decided to try the next fun run, but she didn't want anyone to see her train, so she ran at eleven o'clock at night so no one would see the cottage cheese in her thighs.

She was apprehensive about the race. The night before, she kept getting up and looking at the clock. It seemed like two hours passed between 2 A.M. and 2:02 A.M.

Fran doesn't do things half-heartedly. She ran the race and enjoyed it so much that she decided to enter the prestigious Honolulu marathon. When she finished that marathon, exhausted and sore, she vowed that she would never run another marathon ever again. She ran four more that year.

Running for Fran became not just a way to lose weight and stay in shape. It became both the embodiment and the motivation of her tremendous drive, positive mindset, and purpose. Since her first marathon over twenty years ago, Fran has run twenty-five marathons and hundreds of shorter races. She is currently in the process of running a marathon in every state, as well as Washington D.C. When she has accomplished that feat, she is planning to run a marathon in every Canadian province, and then on every continent.

Her running keeps her focused on other areas of her life. It is her mantra. It helps her in the discipline of having her mind rule her body. Her running is her life. Her running saved her life.

Several years ago, while getting routine medical care following a car accident, her doctor found a mass on her left side. Fran was fit and strong, of course, and weighed 125 pounds at five feet, five inches tall, so her general health couldn't be better. If she was going to have to deal with a medical problem, she had the right physique and spirit. She was going to need all of that physical and mental strength. She was diagnosed with pancreatic cancer.

At first Fran told no one about the diagnosis, figuring that she would get through without the necessity of involving others. But when the doctors in Phoenix told her there was nothing more they could do for her and sent her to Texas, that plan was no longer viable.

In Texas, she was assigned nine doctors, none of whom were optimistic about her chances of survival. The ordeal was turning into a nightmare, and Fran had experienced this bad dream before.

Earlier, in 1981, Stan had received his assignment to Nellis A.F.B. in Las Vegas, Nevada. At the routine physical prior to his promotion as Lt. Colonel, a mass was found. A day later he was diagnosed with seminoma cancer. Within hours he had lost his dream and was given four months to live.

Stan battled hard for survival. He is a spiritual man who in his youth had left the seminary where he was studying to become a Roman

Catholic priest, to join the Air Force. With humor, grace, tremendous drive, and Fran's strength and positive outlook, Stan survived the chemotherapy, the surgery, and the roller coaster of cancer treatment and returned to fly the F-16 Falcon jet.

So Fran knew what it would take to defeat a terminal illness, and she wasted no time in putting that plan into effect, despite the poor prognosis. Or maybe because of the poor prognosis.

On the first day in the hospital she was brought her food in bed. She told the nurses that she had two good feet and was quite capable of walking to the dining hall. Fran subsequently had almost all her meals there. The request to eat in the dining hall shocked the medical staff, but Fran had something even more shocking the next day.

"I asked the doctors whether I could run around the second floor," said Fran.

The second floor had an outside, covered walkway that Fran had earmarked as a place she could run. The doctors were stunned, but Fran was persistent. Fran knew that running was an essential part of her life and taking it away would be devastating. The doctors reluctantly agreed. She headed down to the second floor and started running timed laps.

Eating in the cafeteria, running around the second floor—this is how Fran kept control of her life, refusing to compromise with hospital administration and pancreatic cancer. She also knew that humor was essential. Here, Fran was lucky in that a wonderful lady, Mary Williams of El Paso, Texas, shared her room. The two of them would spend a lot of time laughing and becoming best friends. Mary became Fran's secretary, screening calls and making a variety of elaborate excuses to callers with whom Fran did not want to speak. That was another part of Fran's policy—avoid sympathy cards and anyone who was going to have a negative or fatalistic view.

Despite Fran's refusal to become passive and dependent, despite her humor and her strength, despite her positive outlook and her otherwise healthy body, the disease was progressing. Fran, however, kept the faith.

By faith, Fran is Greek Orthodox, and at this time she received a call from a friend, Imogene Welch. Imogene has been a long-time member of the TOPS board and the organization's Retreat Director. Imogene told her that she had been relocated to Covina, California. Fran immediately saw the connection. Covina was the home of the only Greek Orthodox shrine in North America. This was no chance coincidence.

Without Fran's knowledge, Imogene visited the shrine and met the priest. The priest told her about St. Nectarios, the patron saint of cures for the terminally ill in the Greek Orthodox Church. When St. Nectarios died in 1927, oil emanated from his rib, the priest explained, and this oil has tremendous healing properties. The priest gave Imogene a small amount of the oil and told her to send it to Fran with the instructions to put it on the affected part of her body. He demonstrated this by motioning to the pancreas even though Imogene had never told him where Fran's cancer was located.

When the package from Covina arrived, Fran and Stan knelt and prayed. Then Fran applied the oil to the area around her pancreas.

She's hasn't been sick since.

That was seven years and twenty-five marathons and hundreds of miles run ago.

Her recovery simply reinforced Fran's tremendous sense of purpose. She always runs for charitable causes. Every October she runs the Race for the Cure, a race to help breast cancer awareness. The pin signs worn on the backs of the runners have the names of those who are being remembered in the race.

"On mine I wear IN MEMORY OF ALEXANDRIA CONDO, my mother who died of breast cancer, and IN CELEBRATION OF TESS BEREOLOS, my sister who survived it," says Fran.

Fran has run thousands of miles for other people. She also ran the Olympic torch in Las Vegas prior to the 1984 Los Angeles Olympics. Fran inspires people not only on the road but on stage, too, as a motivational speaker with several powerful messages and valuable tactics for regaining health and living life to the full.

Fran talks about making the most of our time. "What cancer taught me more than anything else is to use time wisely," she says.

Her annual New Year's resolution involves looking at her behavior and eliminating one activity that is no longer rewarding. Recently, for example, she decided that the gourmet group, in which she and Stan were members, had outlived its value so that they decided to stop that activity. They are not waiting until Stan retires from Boeing as an instructor pilot to live their life.

Terrific Tactic

Review your behaviors frequently, and change any which have outlived their usefulness.

Living every moment as if she has just a few months left to live is a philosophy that both she and Stan share.

"Don't be afraid to change. Be a risk taker," advises Fran. "Stan and I are not spectators in life; we are in it," she adds. The couple plans annual adventures and recently went whitewater rafting fifty-five miles through the Grand Canyon and is planning to hike the Canyon, rim to rim.

Two of Fran's principles are relevant to both weight loss and life. "Be prepared," Fran advises. She herself always takes a cooler or sandwich bag—which contains two light yogurts, fruit, a sandwich, and iced water—with her everywhere she goes.

Terrific Tactic

***Be prepared. Anticipate temptations and high-risk situations
by taking healthy snacks with you.***

"Don't let anything get in the way of your goals," Fran says. This
includes age, weight, or other problems. For Fran, it's simply a matter
of deciding to do it. "'I can't' means 'I don't want to,'" she claims.

"I can't" means "I don't want to."

So just how long will Fran continue to run marathons? Heading
into her late fifties, will she soon be hanging up the running shoes?

"I was recently thinking about that question when I was driving to
the National Senior Olympics in Tucson, Arizona. There I ran with an
eighty-six-year-old blind woman. Just because she couldn't see didn't
mean she couldn't run. What an inspiration that was to me. I thought,
I haven't even begun to scratch the surface with my running," says Fran.

Fran will run and live her life with passion, spirit, and purpose. And
all the time inspired by the verse from Hebrews: "Run with Endurance
the Race Set Before You."

Rankin's Reminders

Mind Over Matter

Believe in yourself and your ability to lose weight. Belief is the most important tool you have. Without it, you're lost.

Visualize success. Images have a powerful effect on the subconscious and the body. If you can't imagine success, you can't achieve it.

Maintain positive energy. Energy translates into positive moods and positive thoughts. Exercise is the best way of maintaining high energy levels.

Understand which part of you is destructive to health and weight loss. You have many sides to you. Which parts are healthy and which destructive? Who is doing the destructive eating?

Take control. Assert the healthy side of you; control immature, destructive, and helpless feelings.

Be conscious of your binging. Avoid binge triggers; don't keep binge food at home, and try not to eat alone if you are a binger.

Your body is your unconscious. Find peace—meditate, relax, and laugh.

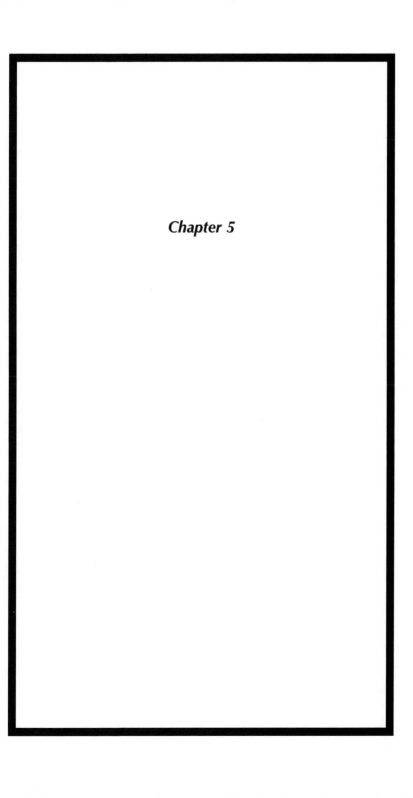

Chapter 5

Owning Up

Take responsibility and give up the illusion of the quick fix

"Take your life into your own hands and what happens? A terrible thing: no one to blame." – Erica Jong

There once was a young Japanese man who wanted to become a Zen master. So he sought out a famous Zen teacher and asked him how long it would take to reach his goal.

"If you study really hard and give me your complete concentration and attention twenty-four hours a day, it will take ten years," said the teacher.

"Ten years!" exclaimed the pupil. "Suppose I really give it everything I have, day and night; then how long will it take?" enthused the young man.

"Twenty years!" replied the teacher.

"No wait, you don't understand. I'll give it everything I have, I'll follow every instruction to the letter; then how long will it take?" asked the pupil.

"Thirty years!" replied the teacher.

"How can this be!" exclaimed the pupil. "Each time I offer to put in more work, you say it will take me longer."

"A man in such a hurry learns slowly," replied the teacher.

Most of us live such fast-paced lives that we learn slowly. We are in a rush and so we focus on the ends rather than the means, taking little time to focus on the process. We look for shortcuts; we delegate as much as we can, including responsibility. Especially responsibility. Responsibility means effort — time-consuming effort.

There is only so much time available, so the less to do, the better. It is not just that we are inherently lazy. It's adaptive to find shortcuts to problems and achieve goals in the shortest possible time. The problem is that some goals benefit from shortcuts, and others do not. If your goal is spiritually meaningless—e.g., fixing your dishwasher—saving time makes sense. If your goal is spiritually meaningful, however, short-cuts won't work because the *pursuit* of spiritually meaningful goals is as important as the goal itself. For example, reducing a religious service to five minutes as a timesaving convenience would render the service useless as a spiritual exercise.

Most of the time we live in a spiritual void. Many activities are mundane and seem to have little real meaning. Technology increasingly allows us to indulge our addiction to convenience. Ironically, the more successful we are at finding shortcuts to trivial goals, the more we are incapable of embarking on more meaningful exercises. Instead of buying more time to pursue more meaningful activities, convenience addiction actually reinforces impatience and low frustration tolerance. Almost all of the valuable aspects of life take time, but few people are prepared to wait.

Health, Spirituality, and Dependence

Our health should have spiritual meaning because it literally is a matter of life and death. But health, too, is sold as a convenience. An exercise program that takes only five minutes a day, a diet where you can eat anything you want, a pill that will dissolve hunger, and surgery that will remove fat are the headline grabbers and sought-after products.

Other factors dilute our sense of responsibility. We have a concept of medicine and health that places the patient in a dependent, subservient, and passive position. The responsibility of the patient in Western allopathic medicine is to simply hand over power to the doctor and let her work her magic. Even worse, with the advent of HMOs many people don't even have much or any say in their choice of physician, let alone their treatment.

So it's hardly surprising that when it comes to health issues, we look outside us for the answers to our problems. We expect others, products, and services to make us okay. We have been trained to take no responsibility.

Looking outside ourselves for the answer to our problems will not work. Not only are we susceptible to fads and frauds, but we are also wasting valuable time that could be spent learning how to take care of ourselves. In addition, we are setting ourselves up for failure.

Nowhere is the cycle of despair more evident than in the area of weight management. A majority of women have tried dozens of weight-loss products. Almost all of the weight-control products do not address the real issues of lifestyle change and, as a result, produce only temporary results at best.

The result is a cycle of repeated failures that have a devastating effect on self-esteem and hope. Research on yo-yo dieting has shown that the main negative effects of continued weight cycling are on the psyche rather than on the body. Quick fixes lead to long-term disrepair—and despair.

Desperation

The approach to weight and weight management in our culture provides unworkable solutions to impossible expectations. Hardly surprising then that so many feel like failures and are desperate for a solution.

Desperation is the mother of delusion. The more desperate we are, the more we need to believe in the answer so that more and more power is projected into purveyed products. As a result, the search for the Holy Grail only grows more intense and more unrealistic.

One of the ironies of the search for the quick fix is that, even if there were one, it wouldn't work. It would not work because, when it comes to making lifestyle changes that are affected by many decisions in the course of a day, a person needs to be in conscious control, completely vigilant—not putting blind faith in some outside force. For example, at various times in the course of my career, desperate smokers have asked me to simply lock them away and drug them for the five days of nicotine withdrawal. Surely, they suggested, this would be the answer to quitting smoking.

It isn't. Not only would the smoker learn no techniques to manage a life without smoking, but the smoker also would see that he had done nothing to create his success. *All magic bullets and quick fixes are defeatist because their implicit message is that the person is powerless to change himself.* They keep us precisely in the wrong corner—dependent and helpless.

Jean Stacy's story about a woman who invests her dreams of thinness into a medical procedure is a classic example of how a lifetime of frustration leads to desperation and delusion. It is tempting to think that as a society we have evolved significantly in the twenty-five years since the main events in Jean's story unfolded, but that, too, is a delusion. Medicine will always be offering techniques and hope to anyone suffering from a physical problem. As the rules are currently constructed, such techniques, including medications, are approved before all of the side effects are known. The surgical bypass operation for which Jean so eagerly signed up was an approved medical procedure. This procedure pioneered the way for today's gastric bypass surgery, which was developed in the light of the consequences and symptoms that Jean reports in her story.

Jean's story captures all too vividly what happens when need collides with promise. The powerful cocktail of primitive emotional drive and the seduction of ultimate success highjack reason. If we are lucky, all we get is a severe hangover—Jean Stacy got a whole lot more. Ironically, at the precise moment Jean was giving up her power and handing over responsibility for her problem, she actually believed that she was in control and taking the initiative.

In Jean's case, even the physicians performing the operation seemingly had some doubts and were not misleading her intentionally or otherwise. Their desire to help the obese was well intentioned and based on the known science of the day. Jean's delusion came entirely from within, as she now freely admits. That cannot be said of the current market environment and the many weight-loss products and services available. Some are downright fraudulent and many, completely unnecessary, if not counterproductive, and even dangerous.

Almost any product can be justified as helpful in weight loss, and is, because of the clever use of the fine print. In almost every weight-loss product promotion there is a man (rarely a woman, you note), delivering a message at almost indecipherable warp factor ten-speed that notes that the product will work "in combination with the appropriate diet and exercise." Print ads are no better, delivering the same message, this time in an almost invisible font size that can be comfortably viewed if you happen to have a good pair of binoculars readily available.

Appropriate diet and exercise *are the active ingredients* of any successful formula, and any activity can be attached to a formula to make it sound like a wonder product. Sleeping two hours each afternoon in a hammock, *in combination with appropriate diet and exercise,* will help you lose weight. Sitting in a tree fifteen minutes each day, *in combination with appropriate diet and exercise,* will help you lose weight. I now wait in confident expectation that some marketing genius will soon introduce the weight-loss hammock and, just maybe, the weight-loss tree house.

What is perhaps more troubling is that the weight-loss hammock might actually be a commercial success because enough people have a combination of a history of failure, low self-esteem, desperation, convenience addiction, and helplessness to actually invest in the ridiculous idea. Each time a person invests in such an idea, she is not just agreeing to fork over $19.95 plus shipping and handling. She is distracting herself from the real issues. She is investing in powerlessness.

How many women and men have embarked on the latest fad with the dream that this is the diet, pill, or program that will finally make the difference? It can take a long time to see through that fantasy; but when you do, you have discovered several powerful and promising messages. There are no shortcuts but many blind alleys.

Irresistible Deception—Jean Stacy

Jean's story shows what happens when you give up responsibility and how hard it can be to wrestle it back from the illusion that there is an external answer to internal problems.

By the time Jean was in kindergarten she was almost the size of some of the sixth graders. She hated being big — mainly tall with a frame to match. She remembers being taken to the nurse's office to be measured and weighed. The first time they did it, she wanted to die. They called out the children's names and weights: "Frank Ozitz — thirty-two pounds; Judy Smith — thirty-five pounds; Jean Stauss (her maiden name) — sixty-three pounds." After that, whenever the teacher announced that the class was going to be weighed, Jean would excuse herself and go to the restroom, then come back, saying she was sick and had to go home. That's how she survived kindergarten.

As Jean was growing up, her weight made her sad, but she never said anything about it or revealed her hurt. Her father never mentioned her weight at all, nor did her brother or sister. Her mother, who was the only other overweight member of the family, also said nothing. Jean and her mother were very close, bonded by their shared love of music— and food.

"I was never put down by my family, just the rest of the world," remembers Jean.

It wasn't that Jean was without friends or that she was a recluse. She got along with everyone, but her nickname, "Steamroller," really hurt. She took dance lessons with her little sister, Carol, in a class of peers where she was always twenty pounds heavier and a head taller than all the others. She would hear people say, "What is SHE doing dancing with all those little kids." SHE was only five.

Unsure if there really was anything that could be done, and not wanting to show her vulnerability, Jean turned to humor as a defense. One time she was appearing in a local city circus, doing a trampoline routine with her sister and a friend. Jean was good once she was on the trampoline, but flipping onto it like the others was impossible. So she was dressed as a clown who stumbled and fumbled her way on. Jean— the perfect clown, laughing on the outside, crying on the inside.

The teenage years were really hard. Jean would watch guys line up at the door, waiting to date her sister. The only guys waiting for her were on the high school football team; they needed someone "big" on whom to practice tackling. Even they came up to Jean's shoulders and were considerably lighter. Undaunted, Jean remained very active. She belonged to a sports club and excelled at volleyball, basketball, and baseball. At five feet, nine inches, she was so tall that she could dominate the net in volleyball, almost dunk the basketball, and was the home-run queen in baseball. The ball would fly forever once she hit it, which was good because she could barely run around the bases.

Jean realized there was little she could do about her height, but she could have done something about her weight. But food was intimately linked to the special relationship she had with her mom. Together, they were the last ones to leave the dinner table because they were busy eating leftovers. Her mother never made small meals.

"We had about ten courses every time. After all, we couldn't WASTE food," Jean remembers.

Jean's family also rewarded her with food—or with money to buy it. She would do almost anything for it. On occasions she would stick her hand into a cage of garden snakes to pull one out for her brother, Bob, who would pay her fifty cents for the feat. And with fifty cents she could get a whole bag of candy.

"I buried myself in goodies," Jean says.

By the time she was a junior in high school, Jean was hanging out with the sailors at the nearby Great Lakes Naval Training Center. At least they were her size and there, for the first time, she felt socially comfortable. Little did she realize at the time how significant this connection with the Navy would be in her life.

The first influence occurred at her senior prom. She had a date with a sailor who was flying in from Norfolk especially for the occasion. She had bought the tickets, the long dress, and the shoes and was so excited to have an escort for her big night. The night before the prom, the sailor's ex-girlfriend broke up with her current beau, and the sailor chose to take her instead of Jean.

"My brother offered to take me, but I could never have faced anyone again, so I just stayed home. This time I wasn't crying on the inside. I was sobbing for everyone to hear," Jean says.

Crushed and humiliated, Jean vowed that night to lose the weight. She started by using her babysitting money to embark on a secret course of diet pills. Then there was the secret course of laxatives, then more pills, and just about every diet of which you've ever heard and some you haven't. Jean was taking so many pills at one point that she could hardly walk straight.

The weight would come off in the short term, and Jean would be ecstatic. It would inevitably return and so did the self-blame and a few extra pounds. When Jean graduated from high school, she weighed 235 pounds. When five years later she met Jim, the man of her dreams, she weighed 265.

"I was amazed he wanted to marry me. How could anyone ever love me?" recalls Jean.

Jim was in the Navy; after a whirlwind romance they were married, and within two weeks Jim was sent to Guam. When he came back eighteen months later, he had a nine-month-old daughter. Two years later there was another daughter.

Jean **lost** weight during pregnancy—about twenty pounds each time. But she couldn't stay pregnant forever. She still needed to do something about her weight.

At that time, the Navy was offering a weight-loss program designed to help new recruits lose weight fast. It was similar to the Atkins diet.

Jean lost sixty-five pounds in a short space of time and was thrilled, until she was told she could not stay on it indefinitely. When she changed her diet the weight all came back, leaving Jean feeling even more like a failure.

And so this is how it was. Each time Jim left for another tour, Jean vowed to lose weight and surprise her husband when he returned, but each time she would fail.

"I felt like a real failure. I couldn't do anything right."

There were constant reminders of this humiliation. Jean couldn't go to San Diego Padre baseball games if it was the least bit cool because she and her jacket did not fit in the same seat. Jean loved walking, especially with her girls, but if she saw teens up ahead she would find an excuse to cross the street so that her kids were not embarrassed by hearing nasty remarks. Turnstiles and revolving doors were a killer, but eating out was the worst.

"I could have gone all day without eating and had a salad in front of me, but I felt like people were staring at me thinking 'There she is—eating again!'"

Humiliation and despair will do that to you.

By this time, Jean was living in Navy housing where she met Nelda, a neighbor. Nelda had also been obese but was losing weight like crazy. She would visit Jean, eat everything in sight, and come back the next day with a five-pound weight loss!

"This was it—God's gift to the fat person!" says Jean.

"It" was an operation called the intestinal bypass that was being performed at the Balboa Naval Hospital in San Diego. The operation involved surgically creating an intestinal bypass so that food simply would not be absorbed into the system.

Anyone who has ever been desperate will know how Jean raced to the Naval hospital to get the details and apply without delay. She had waited her whole life for this moment. At last, she was going to be normal!

She weighed-in at 315 pounds and, because successful candidates had to be more than a hundred pounds overweight, she immediately qualified.

"I wouldn't have to do anything, and the weight would just drop off. This would be easy. A cinch," Jean thought.

Her physician warned her against the surgery, citing the many dangers that were very possible. He sat on his desk and said, "This is very dangerous. All you have to do is to stop eating."

Jean responded. "It's okay for you to say that. You sit there with a skinny body. You simply don't understand."

Understand the lifetime of humiliation and shame. Understand the lifetime of failure. Understand the nature of the food addiction. Understand that for Jean, it was lose weight or die.

The omens for the surgery were not good. Her mother came out to San Diego two weeks prior to the surgery to take care of the children. Her mother, who had diabetes and had lost her husband several years before, was very concerned about the procedure but kept her feelings to herself. She supported Jean in whatever she wanted to do, despite her own anxiety. A few days before the scheduled surgery, her mom felt unwell and went to the doctor. She had had a heart attack.

Her mother refused to let her heart attack get in the way of Jean's surgery. So, having been checked out and put on medication, she was back with her grandchildren as Jean entered the hospital.

The day before the scheduled surgery Jean's physician visited her and once again asked her to reconsider her decision to have the operation. She told him in no uncertain terms to leave.

"I didn't care if I died on the operating table; I was doing something about my weight," recalls Jean.

Jean was scheduled for early-morning surgery, but as the day wore on and she hadn't been taken to the operating room, she started to get very nervous. She couldn't face not going through with it now. By noon, she was really concerned, and when they came to see her at 3:30 she was almost beside herself.

There had been a flood in the operating room, and the surgery needed to be postponed for three days. Needless to say, Jean was disappointed but had no doubts about her choice. After all, this was going to fix her problem for life. She did not change her view when one of the operating doctors visited her and suggested that the delay was an omen and that she should reconsider. She asked him in no uncertain terms to leave, too.

And so on January 20, 1977, Jean had her surgery—the magic bullet, the quick fix.

It has taken her over twenty years to recover from it.

She immediately started with major vomiting and diarrhea—sometimes up to thirty times a day. Rather than leaving the hospital to go home to her family a new woman, Jean was confined to the hospital for months at a time. She had just about every test ever heard about and some just made up. The precise problem could not be pinpointed, so that Jean was sent to psychiatrists for months on end. Despite talk of "psychosomatic illness," the psychiatrists could find nothing wrong with her. Jean knew it wasn't psychosomatic and thought the psychiatrists were fishing for an answer.

She had nine further surgeries, and nothing helped. She was in the bathroom almost constantly. She had three painful bone marrow biopsies. She could keep almost nothing down. BUT she did lose weight. In a macabre testament to the grip of her obsession, Jean recalls feeling good that the hospital gown actually fit her for the first time.

This nightmare continued for years. In 1979 Jean spent five consecutive months in the hospital and was getting worse. That December she pleaded with the doctors to allow her out for Christmas so that she could be with her children. She was desperate and thought she was going to die. The doctors told her that she simply would not be able to survive out of the hospital.

"I'll show you I can," she replied. Eventually persuaded by the fact that there seemed little to lose and by Jean's tenacity, the doctors agreed to let her go for Christmas day.

Jean was ecstatic. And for good reason.

Her whole ordeal had been extremely hard on her husband and her daughters, now in their middle childhood. Jim had to stay in the Navy to ensure that the enormous medical costs would be covered. On several occasions Jim had to make emergency flights home because Jean was in critical condition. On several occasions, Jim was being winched back aboard his ship via helicopter when he received news that he had to return immediately because Jean had taken a turn for the worse.

Her children had to stay with a variety of friends and Navy families while their parents were absent. Their dad would not allow them to visit the hospital and see their mother in such an appalling condition. The children had not seen her for several months. In fact, they did not know whether she was really alive.

Later, her daughter would tell Jean what that trip home for Christmas meant. "I'll never forget that, Mom," said her daughter. "It was only then that I knew that you were alive."

There's a photo taken that Christmas morning of Jean with her kids. It was good that the photographer didn't wait too much longer. By the afternoon Jean was very ill and back in the hospital. They were waiting for her. They hadn't even changed her bed.

The procedures and operations continued—kidney surgery to remove a huge stone, one of twenty-six that Jean passed. Then there was a collapsed lung, biopsies, a burst intestine, and much, much more! Finally, the doctors gave her the news: her only chance to survive was to reverse the bypass. They also told Jean that once the bypass was reversed she would likely gain back all the weight that she had lost—plus more.

How could this happen? This was supposed to be the miracle cure, the easy way. After all she had been through, how could doctors do something to make her fat again? She had gone from 315 pounds down to 160, but she was dying. It just wasn't fair.

So Jean chose dying over being fat again.

When the doctors told her they wanted to reverse the bypass, Jean told them flatly, "Over my dead body." She simply refused to give her consent.

"I wasn't thinking straight. I didn't care about myself," recalls Jean. Looking back or from the outside, one can see the distorted thinking that accompanies desperation. And Jean had invested an enormous amount of time, effort, and faith in the bypass. To give it up would surely be to give up all hope.

Fortunately, the decision didn't rest with Jean now. When she first agreed to the operation, she had signed her consent, allowing the doctors to reverse the operation if they felt it was necessary. It was out of Jean's hands.

As reality was allowed to creep back, Jean felt stupid. How could she have believed it was going to be this simple? She had selectively forgotten about the times she had walked for miles with Nelda while she was passing kidney stones. Or the times she had wrapped Nelda's arthritic feet in warm towels when she was in horrible pain. All she remembered was watching Nelda eat like crazy and losing 228 pounds.

Terrific Tactic

If someone's weight-loss efforts seem too good to be true, don't automatically accept what he says. Investigate further.

What she couldn't have known at the time was Nelda's ultimate fate. Nelda reportedly went from frumpy to beautiful and with newfound self-esteem, went in search of a better life. By the time she was thirty-three, Nelda was dead—from heart, kidney, and liver problems.

In February 1980, Jean's bypass was reversed. Jean was hopelessly depressed. Even after the bypass was reversed, she was still vomiting and spending more time in the hospital than out. It was extraordinarily hard to adjust. When she first had the bypass, she had developed some horrible eating habits because the more she ate, the faster she would lose. She no longer ate one quarter pounder, but two. She'd buy a six-pack of candy and after eating two or three pieces, eat the rest because she didn't want her family to see the evidence of her excesses.

"I LOVED eating. After all, I wouldn't have weighed 315 pounds if I didn't love food," says Jean.

After the bypass was reversed, Jean had to cut way back, but the pounds were still piling on. Even when she was being careful and making reasonable choices, the vomiting still hadn't stopped, and her weight skyrocketed back up to 315. She hated her predicament, and she hated herself.

At this point, Jean's friend, Debbie, introduced her to TOPS. Debbie told her that because she weighed over three hundred pounds she might have to go the feed store to get weighed.

"Not this girl. I had been humiliated for the last time, so I started to cut back BEFORE I joined," Jean says.

When she went to her first meeting a few weeks later in Santee, California, she weighed-in at 282 pounds. But at that first meeting she found more than a scale that could take her weight.

"After all I had been through I didn't expect much, but when I walked into that room, my whole life changed. I was embraced by the most wonderful, caring group of ladies I'd ever met. Many are still my best friends now. And they all had weight problems—I wasn't alone. They understood my frustrations. They had a lot of the same ones—and they cared," says Jean.

Instead of locking her feelings away, Jean now had a group of friends whom she could trust. She wasn't alone. They were all positive, and they could laugh together. Humor instead of tears, rather than humor hiding the tears.

Seeing others being successful restored hope. Learning about sensible approaches reduced her desperation.

"I learned I was not the only crazy one—or crazy at all."

Most of all, the group restored Jean's self-esteem. She realized that she had been way too hard on herself. That she set impossible standards, and when she drove herself into despair she was only left with fantasy remedies. Most of all she learned two things that are essential for success.

"I was worth something again. For the very first time in my life, I realized I was a good person.

"I also realized that it is my responsibility to take control of my life. I can't expect anything or anyone else to do it for me."

Jean's medical problems continued, but with her newfound support and new attitude she could handle them much better. In 1984, after a battery of tests by a gastroenterology research team, the cause of her problems was finally discovered. She had a paralyzed stomach, a rare condition that necessitated the removal of most of that organ. Even then, the vomiting didn't stop. She still ate, even though she spent an inordinate amount of time in the bathroom. But she was making good choices and exercising faithfully. She didn't eliminate any foods completely from her diet but found a way to eat them sensibly.

As her weight was reducing she met with her physician—the same one who had warned her against the operation in the beginning. He was gracious enough not to say, "I told you so," but instead tried to negotiate a goal that was medically sensible. Initially he felt that 235 pounds was a good goal, but she talked him into 190. In 1986 Jean finally reached her goal. She not only reached her goal but she was also the chapter "queen," having lost over ninety pounds.

"I was on cloud nine. It was the first time I felt like a winner," Jean says.

Her health was beginning to deteriorate again, however. She contracted a bacterial infection and had to return to the hospital for fourteen days of antibiotics. She survived that scare, but days later her temperature went over 105, and she was back in the hospital again. This time it was a blood infection. The treatment required her to be packed in ice because of a dangerously high fever. She had convulsions, several seizures, and was critically ill. After three weeks of fever and seizures she was well enough to go home. But three days later the problem returned—she couldn't breathe and had clots in her lungs and brain. After three more weeks of fever and seizures, it was finally over. Later that year she had her final surgery when tubes were inserted in her stomach.

That was twelve years ago. Today Jean is eating and exercising sensibly. Her weight, which increased immediately after her last operation, is currently down in the 230s, but what matters most to Jean is meeting and talking to members, giving encouragement, and sharing—all of which give her hope and purpose and reinforced the positive in her life.

For anyone who wants to listen—and there are many—Jean sounds this warning: "There is no easy way to reduce. There is nothing better than sensible food choices and exercise. If my story will help one person make a sensible choice of weight reduction instead of some 'easy' choice, I will feel I've gone through this hell for a good reason."

Nothing is easier than self deceit. For what each man wishes, that he also believes to be true. – Demosthenes

A Long-Awaited Insight—Ann Brackett

Ann Brackett's search for the magic answer will surely find resonance in almost every contemporary woman. Faced with mounting adversity, Ann finally finds her way to a universal truth. This is her story.

As I reflect on my life, I remember the many times I tried to lose weight. Every time a new diet came out, I tried it. I've eaten cabbage soup for weeks, grapefruit until my mouth was so sore I couldn't eat, and read every book that had a new idea on how to lose weight. And those magazines at the checkout with the wonderful news … lose ten pounds in a week? I bought and read them all! This was the diet that was going to work for me!

I wasn't always overweight. When I look back at pictures from elementary school, I was of normal size. But then the teenage years began. By eighth grade I had reached 160 pounds. I became a "wallflower" because of teasing and embarrassment over my size. I hated physical education, as I was the last one picked for a team. They didn't want "Annie Fannie" on their team. They pointed and laughed at me as I tried to help the team. I just wanted to cry inside. That is where I kept all of my feelings—inside. My family had no idea I was suffering emotionally. As long as I did my chores, did my homework, and was polite, they were happy.

Then I heard some girls talking at school about losing weight by drastically cutting their calories. I decided to do sit-ups and only eat six hundred calories a day. My mother was upset that I was eating so little at meals. In no time, I was at 135 pounds. This new "me" was short-lived and hardly noticed by my classmates. The moment I started eating again the weight started on. In no time I was above 160 pounds.

"Annie Fannie" was back!

I continued to diet over and over again in high school. Each time I started a diet I thought this is the one that's finally going to work, make me thin, and solve my problems. I would start a diet, lose a few pounds, but then not be able to sustain it and would gain the weight back, plus a few more pounds. I just hoped that if I would lose weight and keep it off, I would have dates, go to dances, and do all the things the other girls were doing. Well, it never happened in high school.

I began to hang around with the "wrong crowd." I tried smoking and drinking. I wanted to "fit in" with a group. But after I skipped school one day with my new group my mother put an end to "that group." After receiving a whipping from my mother I was taken to and from school each day. I was not allowed to go to any friend's house. I spent a lot of time alone in my room, dreaming about a different life. I started doing some tutoring at school and volunteering at the hospital to avoid going home.

Then I went off to college with more diets and more dreams! I wanted the people at school to accept me as I was, not judge me by my size and weight. I hoped this school experience would be different. I met a group of girls that I "hung out" with. They were always on diets and always talking of boyfriends. I wanted a boyfriend.

After my second year in college, I met my husband while summering in Maine. I had lost weight. I was back to my 160 pounds and was feeling a little better about myself. At that time I was unaware of my husband's obsession with beautiful bodies. We were both caught up in the romance. I began teaching school. Life was good.

We decided that we would start a family. I started gaining weight quickly. It was OK, as I was eating for two people. For the first time it was all right to be overweight, as I was pregnant. I would lose this weight after I had the baby. Patricia was born. I had gained fifty pounds during my pregnancy. She weighed over nine pounds, but I didn't lose fifty pounds with her birth. So I began going to a weight-reducing group only to find out I was pregnant again, with Judy. Here I was still overweight, with a five-month-old baby, and pregnant. After Judy was born I was up to 220 pounds. Then a week later my Dad died from a stroke.

It was at this time that my husband started nagging me about losing weight. I knew now how he felt about a woman's body. I wanted to please him, and he was supportive in my dieting. So I began yet another diet and then another and another. Weight was down, then up, and then down again. The ever-popular yo-yoing! At this point, my husband just laughed at my attempts. He kept reminding me that I would not stick to it. Each time I would end up weighing more.

I was now up to 240 pounds. Back to Weight Watchers I went. I lost fifty pounds only to find out I was pregnant with Chrissy. I was stressed right out! My Mom was dying from breast cancer, my husband was upset with me, and I was pregnant! Since I had been brought up under the theory, "If you eat you will feel better," I ate!

My mom kept her cancer to herself. She wouldn't talk about it. She had breast cancer that had gone to the bones. Before she went to the doctor she had over a thousand fractures of her bones. Not talking about the cancer made the whole situation almost unbearable. I was teaching school, caring for my Mom before and after school, and pregnant with a child my husband did not want.

When I was five months pregnant my mom died after nine months of extreme suffering. After Chrissy was born my husband kept reminding me what a "slob" I was, how embarrassed he was to be seen with me, and that he would leave me if I didn't lose weight. So more diets, as I was up to 235, until one day in 1990 I just said, "Leave me!" I was so tired of his going out every Friday night alone. He would not take me, as I was an embarrassment to him. I remembered coming home from the hospital after my back surgery only to be told he was going to the Legion Dance. I couldn't believe it! I was miserable! I hated myself and many times wished I were dead. I didn't reach out for help, as I didn't feel I could afford it.

One night after the divorce, as I sat with a bottle of pills, I almost ended everything. But I kept thinking of the girls. What would happen to them? I could go on and make it on my own. I would be able to do it. I had a job, a home, health insurance, and my girls. It was time to be happy.

But to be happy I thought I had to be thin. So off I go to another diet group. I lost weight for a while but then tired of it. I was tired and worried about the finances. I was running the home, teaching school, and bringing up the girls. I had no "me" time.

As I look back now I wish I had had the support of a group. I would have understood the importance of exchange groups and exercise. My daughters would have been brought up in a home with healthy eating habits. We all would have been healthier and happier. But that was not the case. My daughters began having the same weight struggles that I had had.

Then in 1993, Judy, at the age of twenty, was killed in an automobile crash. I couldn't believe it. She had just gone out for a couple of hours with her girlfriends. As the police chief stood in my kitchen, trying to talk to me, it seemed like this must be a bad dream. I must wake up! My heart was broken! I was devastated! I ate and ate to try to comfort myself.

My younger daughter, Chrissy, and I became very close, as Patty was away at college. We traveled and ate out a lot. I did not want to be home. If I was away it was as if it really didn't happen. I tried counseling and praying. It was just so hard to deal with. Until one day, Madelyn Farmer, a colleague at school, asked me to go to TOPS with her. I thought about it. I needed to do something as my blood pressure was up; it was so hard to bend over to talk to my kindergarten students, and I was exhausted all the time. I would give it a try but really didn't expect any great things to happen.

I joined the group in Baileyville, Maine, in January 1995 and weighed-in at 270 pounds. It was a wonderful group of about twenty men and women. They welcomed me with open arms. The program was on the food exchanges. They had contests going on, which they encouraged me to join. I thought I might as well. Then a neighbor, Darald Mitchell, came up to me and started talking. I talked away to him but didn't have a clue who I was talking to, as he had lost over eighty pounds. On the way home, I asked Madelyn who he was, as he seemed to know me. She laughed and said, "That's your neighbor, Mitch." I couldn't believe it! Right then I decided to give it a good try for a month.

At the end of the month I had lost over twenty pounds. I had the best weight loss for the month. During the first year I lost ninety pounds. I wrote everything down in my daily food journal. I kept my calories between 1,000 and 1,200. I tried recipes from the chapter members, began going to workshops, and never missed a meeting. I was eating almost entirely fat free but not exercising.

During 1996 I continued but couldn't seem to get motivated again. The trial came up for vehicular manslaughter against the driver of the car that killed my daughter. The trial brought back all the horror of that dreadful night in August 1993. When could my healing begin? I started emotional eating again. I gained ten, then twenty pounds. I then gained twenty more pounds during the year after having emergency gall bladder surgery.

In 1997 I decided that I was going to add exercise to my program. Others were reaching their goals, but they were walking or using exercise equipment. Maybe this would work for me. So I started walking—first a block, then two blocks, until I was walking miles. Now to get those skis out that had been used once, years before. I was going to learn to cross-country ski. I went on a short ski first before working up to a few miles on the trails at Moosehorn Refuge. I had a great time, and I was losing weight again.

Another motivator was that my oldest daughter, Patty, was being married in July. I wanted to look good for the wedding. I did get down to a size fourteen dress, so was happy. I looked good, but it was an emotional day. My daughter was now on her own, and Judy was unable to be at the wedding. So on comes the emotional eating again. Why couldn't I be one of those people who lose their appetite when stressed?

At the end of 1997 I had to have bladder surgery. I would be unable to do much for six to eight weeks. I was so upset and depressed. The weight was coming on again, and I couldn't seem to stop it. My best friends emailed me or called me and sent many encouraging notes, but I just couldn't get it all together. It just seemed like it was never going to work for me. I was still thinking, "Diet."

Then one day I saw an article, by Barb Hartley in Indiana, about online help, and I decided that I would email for support. The support that I received was wonderful! It is now 1998, and I'm on a roll again, emailing the loop, going to my meetings, doing programs, going to workshops. I am going to do this! I am walking every day, doing food charts, running contests at the TOPS group, sending cards, and doing the exchanges.

I found out about my breast cancer six days before Christmas! I had just gone in for my yearly mammogram. No big deal. Then I get a phone call the next day to return to the hospital for more tests.

I said, "Oh, what did I do, move?"

"No, we saw something."

I just couldn't believe this was happening to me! I became depressed! I felt like Job! Why was my life so full of disappointments and tragedies? What had I done? Was I going to die soon? Could I get through all this?

The most positive event since having my children occurred in the midst of my "cancer ordeal." It was the birth of my granddaughter. Samantha Judith was born just weeks after my diagnosis. What a love! The reason I needed to get on with my treatments and survive. Within the month I had had two surgeries and was preparing for chemotherapy. My TOPS chapter leader, Sandra Pulk, drove me to my treatments in Bangor (a two-hour drive) and worked on my spirit. My school "buddies" made my meals and visited while my principal, Jim Frost, checked on me and prayed with me daily. My teaching partner, Therese McCormick, who was always there to encourage me in my trials, told me to meet the challenge.

"We will get through this! We've been through worse," she said.

I thought, yes, I have been through worse; I have lost a daughter. I CAN do this! So I concentrated on getting through the cancer treatments and getting back to work.

Due to the high risk of infection I was not able to return to my kindergarten classroom for ten months. On comes the weight again by way of that "comfort food." Before the chemotherapy and radiation are over, I am back up to 229. Then while on sick leave it finally clicks! As I'm reading books on healthy eating I remember members in our chapter saying, "This is NOT a diet but a way of life." What I should be concentrating on is eating healthy and being healthy. I began to read *The Choice Is Yours*, use my exchange food chart correctly, drink my water, and walk daily before work. I realized that all of these years I was wanting and expecting some diet to be the answer. The answer wasn't within the diets; it was in me!

I went to my oncologist after my treatments were completed to talk about my taking Tamoxiphen. I was now back on track. The doctor told me that one of the side effects is weight gain.

I told her, "Then I am not taking it!"

"You don't have a choice," she said.

Needless to say I was upset but determined that it was not going to make me gain weight. I knew that there were things that I could do to prevent weight gain. I needed to take charge, to take the responsibility of managing my life and my weight.

I again started writing my daily food down. I balanced my eating with the food exchanges. I began to drink more water. I walked each day and started water aerobics, which lifted my spirits and gave me energy. Finally, I had the answer to my problem. *It was my problem and my solution.*

In the summer I traveled to different parts of the country to meet with my buddies who had supported me via email when I was in desperate need of support. I shared some of the "little tricks" that worked for me: using smaller plates and bowls, dividing food left over when eating out into a takeout container or loading it with pepper, eating slivers instead of big pieces, doing your food chart each day; but, above all, attend those meetings!

T e r r i f i c   T a c t i c

Use small plates and bowls to control portions and your expectations of what is a reasonable amount to eat.

I ended the summer with a seven-and-three-quarter-pound loss. I now have lost 115 pounds and have reached my goal. What a wonderful feeling! It has been a lifetime getting there! And a whole lifetime to realize that eating healthy should be a way of life, not just a diet. Now to go out and "light the way" for other members to reach their goals. Any goal can be reached if you have faith and believe in yourself.

Character—the willingness to accept responsibility for one's own life—is the source from which self-respect springs. – Joan Didion

Stubborn Resistance—Maureen VandeValk

Maureen VandeValk reminds us that others can motivate, cajole, and support; but in the end, the only person who counts is you.

Most of my early childhood memories were usually centered around food. I come from a family with a good strong Scottish background, and both my grandparents and parents had boarders stay in their homes. As a result, there was always a lot of food around. The aroma of homemade bread still brings back pleasant memories of childhood, of a house where even today you cannot enter without being offered a "cup of tea," which is usually accompanied by a table filled with delicious, fattening foods.

I was the youngest of five children, of which four of us had weight problems. The fifth one was a tomboy and very active in sports. I can remember in the summertime, when children in the neighborhood would get together for a game of baseball, always being the last one chosen for a team because I was such a klutz. It soon became more enjoyable to stay indoors, watching TV, reading, or helping my mother to bake. When in elementary school, we would have to go to the school nurse for our health checkup, which included getting weighed. I can remember the feeling of dread when taking home a paper where I was classified as "obese."

When I was thirteen years old, I tried to find a dress to fit me for my oldest sister's wedding, and I had to look in the ladies department. That set a precedent for the rest of my life. Because of my weight I was very self-conscious and shy all through school. I never had a date and was always quite hurt to overhear comments about my size. I was still the second smallest in my family, as I had two older sisters and a brother who were much more overweight than I.

When I graduated from high school I weighed two hundred pounds. In order to enter nurses training, I brought my weight down to 170 pounds by practically starving myself. The two years I was in training, I returned to the two hundred pounds. As a nurse I lived with two other girls. One was very thin, barely weighing a hundred pounds, and the other was always trying to lose twenty pounds. The three of us worked the evening shift, and it soon became our routine to get off work at 12 P.M. and eat a heavy meal, stay up half the night, and sleep most of the day. I can remember one of our "diet attempts"—coming home to have a salad and then exercising so much that I was in agony trying to walk the next day. With this effort I lost sixty pounds but put it back on once I stopped exercising and resumed eating.

After two years I moved back home. My weight was 220, and up to this point, I was still very shy and self-conscious. I was twenty-one and had never had a date. One of my sisters introduced me to my future husband, Joe. I brought my weight down to two hundred pounds for our wedding, mostly by starving. Once we were married I found that I loved to bake and cook for my husband and myself. My weight began to climb, and it took us three years to have a child. My weight at the beginning of the pregnancy was two hundred and at delivery, ninety pounds heavier. I had a daughter two months premature, and I was at the point where my kidneys were ready to shut down. I had toxemia, very high blood pressure, and was retaining fluids. Two weeks after my daughter's birth I lost seventy pounds of fluid. Luckily we had a healthy daughter.

My weight began to climb again, and our hopes for a large family were beginning to disappear. In 1985 (I now weighed over three hundred) I decided to follow my brother's footsteps and have a gastroplasty. *I didn't think I could lose the weight and thought that this procedure would do it for me.* At first it did. I lost over a hundred pounds through this procedure. I became pregnant soon after, however. My weight was 170 pounds at the beginning of my pregnancy and up to two hundred at delivery. I had to have an emergency cesarean section and delivered a healthy baby boy. We were told after this by our doctor that we shouldn't have any more children. I can remember the anesthesiologist making a snide remark about my size when he came to see me before surgery.

For the next three years I was a happy housewife and mother who was growing and growing. During my second pregnancy I had started eating more frequently than three meals a day to be sure that my baby was receiving proper nourishment, and I continued to do so even after he was born. I never had enormous meals but was a constant picker between meals and loved homemade bread and sweets and junk food. My weight soon rose to over three hundred again. My stomach stretched to a point where I could eat large meals again. This combined with eating between meals soon nullified my gastroplasty.

When my baby was three years old I was diagnosed with breast cancer and had to go through a series of radiation and chemotherapy treatments. At this point, my daughter was in grade five, and when I attended one of her parent-teacher meetings I opened her up to ridicule from her classmates because of my size. However, she chose to not tell me but told my mother instead. When I heard about what had happened I became very reluctant to attend similar meetings and events. I soon was staying at home, only going out for groceries and doctors' appointments. Through all of this I was "happy," smiling as if everything was wonderful. My weight kept climbing, and my body would ache at the least bit of exertion. In the summertime, I felt like a beached whale in the heat.

My husband was terrific. He was concerned about my health and my weight, but he never nagged me or put me down because of my size, which is good because I am very stubborn, and that would not have worked. In August of 1996, however, I received a phone call from my brother, Brian. He had also gained back all of the weight that he had lost, plus more, from his gastroplasty. He proceeded to talk to me as no one else would, with sensitivity, for fear of hurting my feelings. He pointed out how much my family loved me and that they didn't want me to die, but if I didn't do something about it now, I wouldn't be around to see my children grow up! I really thought about what he had said and the next day made an appointment to see my doctor. She was surprised when I asked to be weighed, as I usually tried to avoid it during regular appointments. I was shocked to see that my weight was 325 pounds. I asked for her to arrange for me to see a dietitian. I had to be put on a waiting list, so I halfheartedly tried to put myself on a 1,200-calorie diet. But I found myself slipping back into my old eating habits.

On October 21, 1996, things changed dramatically for me! I had my husband take me to the outpatient department of the hospital, thinking I was having a gas attack. I figured they would send me home with a bottle of antacids. Instead I ended up in the intensive care unit, having a pacemaker inserted. The radiation I had gotten for the breast cancer had caused deep scar tissue in my heart, and my heart finally couldn't deal with both that and my heavy weight! The terror I saw on my husband, Joe, and my children's faces finally wakened me to what I was doing to us ALL. I think back now and realize how much in denial I was about myself! It's amazing how you can look at yourself in a mirror and only see your messy hair and not see your size!

I had my mind seriously made up that I was going to lose the weight. I took the first steps I needed in order to regain control over my life. I decided to stay on the 1,200-calorie diet, and I started to write down every bite I ate. I have had so many arguments with myself about food! I would catch myself sneaking a bite of something fattening, and *I soon came to realize that the only person I was hurting was myself.* I began reading labels and choosing foods more wisely. By the end of 1997, I had lost over one hundred pounds.

When I had lost my first fifty pounds, I decided that it was time to start exercising. I would get my husband to drive the kids and me to our local college track, and we began our walking. At first I could barely make it around the track one time, but eventually we were going around at least twenty times. My daughter and I now make a point of walking five miles at least six times a week. We have even walked on

Christmas Day and New Year's Day. When we first started we decided not to make excuses, regardless of the weather conditions. My first winter walking, I minded the cold, so when my husband asked me what I wanted for Christmas, I said an Air Walker. This was set up in front of the TV in the living room, so I had no excuse to skip my daily walk. I now feel that I don't walk for the exercise but because I enjoy it so much. My body has adjusted to the cold, and I've learned how to layer my clothes so that I'm more comfortable in the winter.

Terrific Tactic

**Enlist the support of others to get started on
an exercise program.**

In the three years it took me to lose nearly 180 pounds, I faced some pretty tough challenges. I soon learned after starting my "diet" that it takes a complete change in my lifestyle. I had to change not only my eating habits but also my attitude toward exercising, and learn to drink at least eight glasses of water daily.

Terrific Tactic

**Drink at least eight glasses of water daily. Have water at
every meal and sip throughout the day.**

The biggest change had to be in my mental approach. I had to realize that I couldn't lose the weight for my family—I had to do it for myself. I had to realize that I only hurt myself when I slip. I'm the one to gain the weight—not my family—when I eat something fattening. However, I've also realized that I can't have sweet stuff around me at home. Luckily my family is willing to do without this to help me. They have been wonderful throughout the last four years. When they see me weakening, they talk me out of it and make me stick to my routine.

I've had a recurrence of the breast cancer, which required surgery and two follow-up operations. I am so pleased to say that I didn't have to miss any of my TOPS meetings. Happily, I am cancer free since April 1997. I have been told by my cardiologist that I don't have to worry about my pacemaker failing me before it is time to change the battery. This is because my heart is so much stronger now, and I hardly ever need it to help. I've regained my health and improved it tenfold.

Now my daughter, Mary Jo, and I support each other in our healthy lifestyle efforts. We keep a daily menu on our refrigerator and find this to be a great help. When we see what we've eaten at the end of the day and how many calories we've had, it's easier to say no to anything else.

Terrific Tactic

Keep your food chart or journal on the refrigerator where it is a visible reminder of what you have eaten and your goal.

I have kept in close contact with my doctor, and she does periodical blood-work checks to make sure that I am getting proper nourishment. She has me on a daily multivitamin and on extra calcium. Two years ago I decided to go back to work and am now head cashier in a department store.

For almost my entire life I've been trying to make myself invisible. Now I'm working with the public every day. I have so much more confidence in myself, I can even speak at a public meeting and address

Secret Revelation—Duane Russell

Duane Russell describes the moment that he understood the meaning of responsibility.

I drove up and stopped the car. I looked around to make sure I hadn't been followed. The place seemed quiet, but appearances can be deceptive. Checking all around me I slowly got out of the car. I silently shut the door and then shuffled as quickly as I could toward the building.

I had told Joe I was coming, but he had been sworn to absolute secrecy. I didn't want anyone around. I had already threatened him with serious bodily harm if he ever divulged that I had been there. I think he thought I was joking, but I wasn't. This meant more to me than anything. It was a matter of life or death.

When I entered Joe started to acknowledge me, but he stopped mid-sentence as soon as he saw the determined expression on my face. He turned his eyes away and nodded for me to go inside. I scurried past him.

I could feel my heart pumping and the sweat breaking out all over my body. My body. That is why I was there.

My heart beat faster now, and I felt almost dizzy. It was the moment of truth. I stepped forward and put all of my weight on those cattle scales. I wanted to get off there before anyone should find me, so I barely had time to check the weight. I did see it. Boy, did I see it. Loud and clear. Four hundred and ten pounds.

I left quickly, only half stopping to threaten Joe again if he ever divulged anything about the incident. I got back to the safety of my car. As I leaned forward against the steering wheel, resting my head in my hands, I knew I was headed for a lot of sickness, disease, heart trouble, stroke, or even death. It was painful, but it was the truth. I had opened myself up and had asked for Divine help. I might not like what I was hearing, but I knew it to be true. And as I sat there in the parking lot of the cattle feed store, God gave me another insight.

My mother is not the cause of my obesity, my father is not the cause of my obesity, and something bad in my past is not the cause of my obesity. I—and I alone—am responsible for the person I have become.

I left that parking lot and drove off into the future. We are today what we chose to be yesterday. We are going to be tomorrow what we decide to be today. I had decided then what I wanted to be tomorrow. That tomorrow is here, and I am over one hundred pounds lighter and even lighter in my spirit.

There is hope for me, and there is hope for you. I have been disappointed, discouraged, dissatisfied, desperate, depressed, and even despondent but never defeated. My hope came that day when I let go of control and handed it over to God. He answered my prayer that day and gave me so much more than I could have imagined.

Action springs not from thought, but from a readiness for responsibility. – Dietrich Bonhoeffer

Taking Time to Travel the Distance—Barb Cady

Barb Cady reminds us that the real competition in weight loss—
as with life—is with ourselves.

I have found that time is my greatest ally and worst enemy in my battle to lose weight. There have been times just prior to an important social event that I have panicked and rushed to lose twenty pounds in two weeks. I know better than to do that now, but in the past I have thrown away the prescription for sensible weight loss. Although starvation on occasion did produce a big weight loss, this good fortune was quickly reversed when I re-hydrated. Even worse, more weight came back, leaving me heavier and even more depressed.

There were times when I was doing this that I knew it wasn't really going to work. I wasn't changing my core habits. I knew I couldn't sustain it, and I would soon be back to old habits. I never did admit to myself that once I was "off the diet," not only would my old habits resume, but I also would eat as if I had been trapped on a desert island for months with no food. But, I told myself, I simply don't have "time" to do it "right." I wanted the "quick fix."

Taking the time to make small changes in the way I eat and increasing my activity gradually through time really does work. I have accepted that fact now, even though I don't like it. Exercising self-control means that I will experience some degree of hunger. Maybe it won't be ravenous hunger, but it will still be there in the background nagging, "Feed me!" I don't like that fact either, but it's still true.

Terrific Tactic

Learn to deal with hunger. With persistence, you will learn to control your response to it.

Food was one of my favorite coping mechanisms. I found that I used it in a huge number of ways in many situations. I had to find other tools to take food's place. Through time I became more aware of the role food plays in my life. I discovered that I ate when happy, when upset, for comfort, for joy, out of boredom, when angry, when tired. There is much more involved than just eating less and moving more. Food is plentiful ammunition, and the triggers fire easily. It has taken time and personal honesty to find different ammunition and a less sensitive trigger! Changes I have made have impacted friends, family, and associates, and so I have learned to be more aware and sensitive. I have learned to communicate more openly and effectively. I have learned persistence. And not a moment too soon, I have learned patience.

Terrific Tactic

Find ways other than eating to deal with emotions and fatigue.

Patience and perseverance help with many of life's adventures. Recently I had an opportunity to do some hiking in the mountains with some good friends and acquaintances. Our destination was the largest tree on this continent, a magnificent Sequoia high on the

184

mountaintop. The climb was definitely uphill and steep at times. It tested my abilities and resolve. I had committed to the journey, however, and this made returning to the vehicles in the parking lot a difficult option. However, there were moments when I thought of sliding back down the mountain anyway—it would certainly have been the easier course. But if I had turned back to what was comfortable and known, I would have denied myself a breathtaking experience. I chose to travel the distance.

As our small group hiked, I found it important to go at my own pace. If I tried to keep up with the pace of the group leaders I found myself huffing and puffing, missing the view, and thinking about the parking lot. I reminded myself that this was not a race. I sharpened my focus. I knew I had the strength, stamina, and ability to go the distance to the beautiful tree as long as I went at my own pace. By simply putting aside time constraints and persisting, I freed myself to achieve all that I desired. There are times when being "first" is important, but this is not one of those times. This was not a competition; it was a completion.

"This was not a competition; it was a completion."

Others on the journey encouraged, expressed concern, commiserated, and continued with me. We changed positions as we traveled up the mountain and as our bodies required. It was much easier to go the distance because others were similarly committed to making the trip and understood the process. Stopping, regrouping, reassessing, moving on. Each step brought all of us closer to the tree—our benchmark of progress.

I don't know what would have happened if any one of us had decided to turn around. Would others have followed? Or would we have encouraged the person to stay the course? This option was never verbalized. Because each of us was dedicated, focused, and committed to the journey, we enabled each other to complete the climb with each footstep that echoed on the trail.

The tree was a wonder! What satisfactions to explore its size, sit in its coolness, stand in its center, and be surrounded by its strength and endurance. Scarred by the fires of time, it stood quietly proud and beautiful. It was rejuvenating! Even knowing that the journey was not over and the grade would still occasionally be steep did not diminish my joy and sense of accomplishment.

The remaining distance was covered with a lightness of footfall and spirit that was astounding. Doing the right thing—no matter how difficult—is its own reward. I celebrated, laughed, and began to formulate new challenges while winding my way down the mountain. No one ever said the journey would be easy—only that it would be worthwhile.

In the long run, we shape our lives and we shape ourselves. The process never ends until we die. And the choices we make are ultimately our responsibilty. – Eleanor Roosevelt

Rankin's Reminders

Developing Responsibility

It's up to you. Don't imagine that anyone or anything else can lose weight for you.

Be informed. Find out as much as you can about nutrition, exercise, weight loss, and your own body.

Be active in your health care. Ask questions.

Buy smart. Invest in products that are aimed at helping you help yourself, not making it sound easy.

Genetics are not an excuse. I'm sorry if you think you have the wrong genes, but that doesn't stop you from taking responsibility for being the healthiest you can be.

Don't be afraid of hard work. Lifestyle change is not for wimps.

Put down the gun. There's no magic bullet.

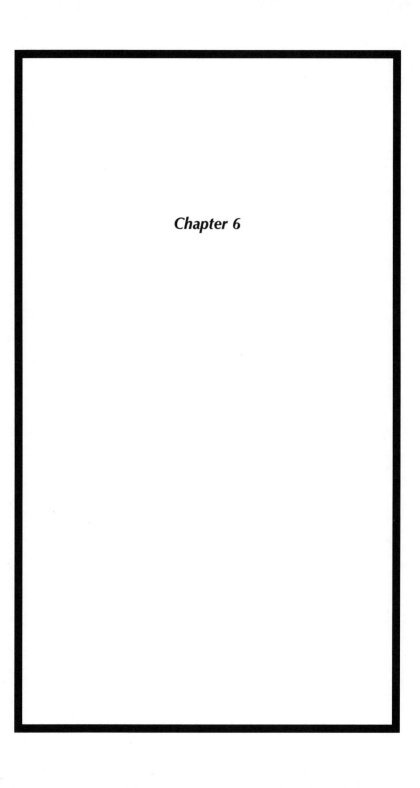

Chapter 6

Priority and Passion

Develop the commitment that is necessary for maintainable weight loss

Work like you don't need the money, love like you've never been hurt, dance like nobody's watching. – Satchel Paige

---

Lifestyle change requires commitment and passion. One of the reasons that many fail at weight loss is that they simply do not make it a high enough priority in their lives and embark on the process halfheartedly.

Passion is the upside of obsession. Obsession means worry, negative preoccupation, and repetition of unhelpful behaviors. Passion means determination, commitment, and a positive drive to meet set goals. An obsessed person gets on the scales three times a day. A passionate person is constantly thinking about how to ensure that when she next gets on the scales she has succeeded.

Goal setting is important for commitment. You can't be committed in a vague way. You have to be committed to specific courses of action and determined to meet tangible goals. Goals should be expressed as specific behaviors, not outcomes. For example, "I am going to eat no more than thirty grams of fat per day" is a better goal than "I am going to lose five pounds." Ideally goals should be set within a time frame: "I am going to exercise for thirty minutes a day this week." Goals should also be written down so that there's no confusion later about exactly what the goal was.

Successful people have very defined, objective goals. Debbee Sereduck started out by setting specific behavioral goals and addressing one behavior at a time. This enabled her to pursue one behavior change whole-heartedly. The strategy worked well for her—she lost more than two hundred pounds. Too often people take a shotgun approach and attempt to change all their unhealthy habits at once. It is difficult to make them all a priority.

Passion and commitment manifest themselves in various ways. Loren Kelly's passion initially manifested itself as a desire to find out as much as he could about nutrition, fitness, and weight loss. Knowledge is power, and it is much easier to be committed and driven if you know not only what you should be doing but also why.

All of the people featured in this section used the power of the group and the support of other people to keep their drive and commitment going. It is not just the support that helps. *Revealing personal goals and going public is the best way of reinforcing commitment.*

Social psychology research shows that while going public is the best way to make a commitment, there are other ways of making commitment tangible. One way is to create a contract that clearly defines changes in specific behaviors and sets what steps will be taken to effect these changes. Signing such a contract then reinforces commitment.

As you read the stories that follow it might be tempting to conclude that the people featured here have determined personalities and that it is these genetic traits that drive them. While that may be true to some degree, it is also true that nearly all of these people were at one time lethargic, uncommitted, and completely indifferent or even fatalistic about their weight. Once each of them was motivated to actually do something about her weight, her commitment was total. Anybody can become passionate. Commitment is not discriminating.

Commitment implies persistence, a behavior that is critical to success in any endeavor. It is easy to keep any behavior going when being successful. The real trick is staying committed when the pounds are not dropping, when a plateau is reached, or when the scales are going north instead of south. Adversity is the true test of commitment.

At the difficult times the committed person doesn't slack off or stop his program; he redoubles his efforts. He goes to more meetings, seeks extra support, and increases his exercise regimen. For the committed and passionate person failure is not an option. Any particular week may not produce the desired weight loss, but overall the people featured here knew that they were going to succeed eventually.

Loren Kelly describes how his commitment led him quickly into a repetitious exercise routine. Because of this determination and the rapid development of the routine, he soon moved from exercising to avoid illness to exercising because it was intrinsically rewarding. Developing new habits requires repetition. The more repetitive the behavior, the quicker it becomes a way of life.

All of the people featured here exude an aura of confidence and commitment that in itself is reinforcing. Others see this level of commitment and expect it. This aura of confidence and determination then becomes another public statement that reinforces commitment. Once you are seen as passionate and determined, it is difficult not to be.

Moreover, the more effort you put into an endeavor, the more you are invested in it.

The harder you work, the harder it is to surrender.
— Vince Lombardi

When determination and commitment are conveyed, they signal to others that you are serious about your weight loss. That doesn't mean that others will necessarily respect your goals and passion, but they will know that you have them. Determination means not letting anything or anyone deflect you from your goals. As you read these stories, it will become apparent that each person enlisted the right support and asserted herself with those who were potential saboteurs. Understanding the threats to your commitment and actively doing something to defuse those threats is another key to success. Those threats will come directly from others and from your own inability to manage time.

Even committed people have bad days. Their drive and determination help them get through the tough times. In fact, the tough times are very often what breed determination and commitment.

Determination—Debbee Sereduck

Debbee's early weight-loss efforts were designed to please her mother. When she realized that she had to lose weight for herself, she settled into a comfortable acceptance of her weight and herself. That changed one day when watching an afternoon talk show.

Despite the fact that no members of my immediate family have a weight problem, it seems that I have always been fat. As a young, fat child I was teased at school. My elementary school companions told me that I would break the jungle gym equipment or would yell "earthquake" when I jumped off of it. It wasn't just that I was fat. I was very tall, and this made me stand out even more.

My elementary school years must have been difficult, but I don't remember them as such. My nine-month-old sister died of what is now called Sudden Infant Death Syndrome when I was in preschool and about two-and-a-half years old. In the first grade I fell off a horse and injured myself badly. In second grade I broke my arm. My parents separated about this time, and I must have had a difficult time because I had to repeat second grade. Now I was older and even bigger than my classmates.

Overall, however, my weight didn't stop me. I was a very active child, a tomboy who water-skied and rode horses. I took the attitude that if people were going to be mean to me, I didn't need them. Although I was occasionally depressed, I was very resilient. My mother had to work long hours to support us, so I took care of some of the house chores and had the responsibility of taking care of my brother, Thomas, five years my junior. I didn't feel sorry for myself at all.

When I was about nine or ten, my mother took me to a Weight Watchers group held in Sears. I really didn't participate or lose any weight, but it marked the first of my mother's attempts to help me lose weight. She was much more concerned about my weight than I was.

My dad's advice was simply, "Don't eat." My mother's efforts were much more intense. She brought in healthy food. She offered me all sorts of rewards to lose weight. Only if I wanted to, she would put me on various diets, shots, pills, and schemes. The reality is that I was okay with my weight. I had lots of friends, both boys and girls. I was active, and I felt pretty good about myself.

By the time I was eighteen my mother had remarried, and both she and my stepfather would do anything to help me lose weight. Their ultimate attempt to help me lose weight was enrolling me in an expensive program of aversion therapy, being conducted at the Schick Center in Encino, California.

In this therapy a counselor sat with me and then gave me some of my favorite tempting foods. The counselor would then get me to chew the food while pointing out all the bad things about the food. Then I would get electric shocks as I was eating it. If the idea was to create a negative association in my mind with that food, it didn't really work. For a couple of weeks, my desire for the food dulled a little but before long it returned with a vengeance.

After the Schick Center episode I realized that I was okay with my weight. My worst feelings at this time did not come from being overweight but from letting my mother down. I could see how much my losing weight meant to her, but it obviously didn't mean that much to me. I just couldn't do it.

Soon after graduating high school I was married to an alcoholic, abusive man. By the time I had my first child I was 250 pounds. I was also scared. I didn't know how to handle my husband's anger. After one particularly violent night, spent avoiding knives hurled in my direction, I knew I had to leave as much to protect my daughter as anything else.

I went home to live with my mother and to get my life back

together. Eventually I met up with a former schoolmate and boyfriend, and we were married. When my second child was born I weighed three hundred pounds. My third and last child was born two years later, and I was 350 pounds. My domestic situation became very difficult after my husband was badly hurt in an accident at work and became dependent on prescription medicines.

At the age of twenty-seven I thought this was how God had intended me to live my life—overweight but healthy. I never let my weight get in the way of being an active mother. I was enthusiastically involved in the local Girl Scout group, which had outings every other weekend. I've always had high self-esteem and would do whatever I had to do to get the job done. So when I caught myself yelling at my children, and I saw how the tension in my marriage was affecting my treatment of the children, I decided I had to leave.

My weight continued to rise, and by the time I met and married Anthony I was at my highest weight. He was wonderful, supportive, and accepting, and I knew he wouldn't be harassing me about my weight.

In 1992 my cousin asked me to go to TOPS. I had no clue what that was, but we checked out a couple of chapters before joining one in Veradale, Washington.

The group seemed great, and having meetings on Monday nights worked well for us. At the first meeting we had to weigh-in. My cousin and her friend went first. I followed and got on the scale. The weight recorder, Jan, kept moving the weights higher—250, 300, and finally, 350—as far as the scale would go but not far enough to weigh me!

I was in tears. Jan said not to worry, but that was a hard thing to do. Jan assured me that she would locate a place for me to weigh and the other members wouldn't have any knowledge of it. After the meeting I didn't tell anyone, not even my husband. That should have told me in itself that I needed to be there.

Jan called me the next day and said she had arranged for me to weigh on the bushel barrel scale at the local grocery store. I went, having no idea how much my weight had increased over the years. I was completely devastated when the scale balanced at 366 pounds.

The first week I tried so hard but still gained weight. Jan encouraged me not to give up. After four or five weeks of not losing weight, I started finding excuses to stay home and not weigh-in at all. After I ran out of excuses I just quit. My cousin and her friend continued to go to TOPS, lost weight, and kept me informed with the latest news of the group.

In June the following year I was motivated to lose weight. Things had been going well in my life, so I thought I would try losing again. I called Jan and set up a time to go back to Yoke's (the store) and weigh. Much to my surprise my weight was even higher than before—378 pounds.

I know now that I set myself up to fail, but at the time I didn't know. I thought that since things were going so good in my life, and my clothes were kind of feeling looser, that I was losing weight. In reality, however, my mind was playing tricks on me because I wanted to lose the weight so badly.

I had been subbing as a school bus driver, and the kids were mercilessly rude about my weight. Some of my coworkers were prejudiced because of my weight.

I never drove any bus without a seat belt, but there is one particular bus that is very old. When I had to drive that bus, I would go out half an hour before I needed to leave to get the seat belt out to stretch it over my lap to buckle it. It was so tight that once I was in it, I didn't undo it until I was done driving for that run. After driving that bus the tops of my legs were so red and bruised from the seat belt cutting into them, and they would hurt for days. But I loved my job, and I wasn't going to let anything stand in the way of it. I'm a good driver, and I love kids.

During the holidays that year, I was watching *The Maury Povich Show*. He was interviewing an obese woman with serious health problems. I immediately thought that I didn't want that to happen to me. I wanted to see my kids grow up and continue to lead an active life.

Something inside me definitely clicked while watching that show. It was then, probably for the first time, that I decided I needed to do something about my weight *for me*.

At first I didn't know what I was going to do or whether I would be successful. I can be very single-minded and determined. I made the decision to focus on just one behavior at a time and give that all my attention. I figured that trying to do everything at once would over-whelm me.

Terrific Tactic

Focusing on one behavior at a time is an excellent strategy. Trying to change everything all at once is a set-up for failure.

The first thing I addressed was being aware of what I was eating. Then I focused on not having second helpings. Once I had this under control, I directed my attention to actual portion sizes. This was a new experience, and I soon realized why I had gained so much weight. I always thought that a portion was the size of a large serving spoon. I had no clue that a serving spoon holds two or three servings. I had to learn to read labels and pay attention to serving sizes. Most of the time it's one-half cup, which is not much.

So I would fix my plate and eat out in the living room while the rest of the family could eat anything and could have as much as they want-ed. It was hard to eat just one serving. So after I was done eating, I wouldn't go back into the kitchen. I set my plate on the counter and got ready to go for a walk with my husband. My children learned how to put the food away and clean up the dishes. This broke two habits I didn't know I had. One was cutting up the children's food and taking a bite here and there. Another was eating leftovers, which I couldn't "let go to waste." (It went to my "waist," but I didn't realize that at the time.)

Avoid dealing with leftovers. Put them away before eating or have others deal with them.

Now that I realized I had to be accountable for my weight, I rejoined the TOPS group and weighed-in each week. I knew I needed more than the scales. I knew I needed to be accountable to others. Because of the group members' caring and understanding, I felt I could trust them to be my monitors. Going public in this way was scary, but I knew I had to do it.

I continued to focus on systematically changing my behavior. For example, I changed my intake to twelve hundred calories and fifteen grams of fat per day. I changed my nighttime snack of Oreo cookies to one of fresh fruit. I never exercised before, but I started using my stationary bike. I don't like exercise any more now than I did before, but I do know that I can't keep my weight off without it.

At first I just sat on the bike and told myself I needed to do this. After a week of talking to myself, I began to ride it very slowly. I set the bike for one hour. I didn't ride it for an hour; it just took that long to convince myself I had to ride it. I would sit there even when I was tired; I'd rest awhile then start riding again. It wasn't long before it was easy to do. I also would go for a walk in the evening after dinner with my husband, and each night we would walk farther, until we could walk anywhere. It got to the point where if I needed one or two things from the store, we would walk or ride our bikes instead of drive. We have a beautiful trail near our house, and as a family we would go for bike rides. When the weather was bad outside, I would exercise to tapes.

Walking after meals, especially the evening meal, is a great strategy that removes you from the kitchen and further temptation, as well as stimulates metabolism.

One of my goals was to square dance. When I got under two hundred pounds we took lessons, five nights a week. Now we are club presidents and have become very involved.

My program became my passion. It had top priority in my life. I knew if it didn't, I wouldn't have a life.

Gradually I reached the small goals that I set for myself. The more I accomplished, the better I felt. I soon realized that my healthier diet and lifestyle were not just good for me but also for the whole family.

I stuck with it with dogged determination. I would not be deterred. If I had a bad day I would refuse to let it get me off track. I trusted my group and attended religiously. I made it an obsession because it had to be.

"I made it an obsession because it had to be."

At my highest weight I weighed 414 pounds. I now weigh 185 and feel great. Family time now consists of square dancing, bike rides, walks, swimming, and other outdoor activities instead of watching television. Shopping for clothes was a chore I hated; now I love to shop. Just knowing I can go into ANY shop, whether I like it or not, and they will have my size. WOO YEA! I can wear my mother's clothes, my kids' clothes, and my best friend Renee's clothes too! I haven't been able to wear her clothes since we were ten years old.

I continue to work at maintaining my lifestyle and weight. If I have learned anything, it is that if you want something badly enough you will never let anyone or anything stand in the way of achieving your goals. Never give up!

> *Take the first step in faith. You don't have to see the whole staircase, just take the first step. — Martin Luther King*

The Scales of Justice—Loren Kelly

Loren describes a remarkable voyage from depression and lethargy to complete fulfillment.

Loren Kelly is an immensely energetic man. Not that it was always like that. For a while he was an immense, lethargic man. It is difficult seeing him now, passionate and driven, and imagine him as anything else. But there was a time when Loren could barely breathe, when sleep apnea had him falling asleep at the wheel, when narcolepsy was more of a reality than alertness.

In those days, he had to wear an air mask to bed; it was hooked up to a breathing apparatus so that he wouldn't expire in the night. Even then sleeping was difficult. No Rapid Eye Movement (REM) sleep meant no dreaming. Good thing, really, because Loren had nothing to dream about, just nightmares.

That was back in the dark days when Loren's obesity meant aches in almost every part of his body, when his back hurt so much he wanted to sit down; but when he sat down he feared he might break the chair. Indeed, at over three hundred pounds, he did break many chairs. This was back in the dark days when Loren refused to look at himself—no photos, no mirrors, no self-esteem.

Then Loren worked in the criminal justice system as a probation officer. To Loren, however, there was little justice in this system. A female supervisor refused to give him a required performance appraisal evaluation, and Loren lost any chance of pay raises. When he received his first paycheck of the year this supervisor walked into his office, threw his paycheck on his desk, laughed, and said: "Here's the big bucks! Get rid of some of that weight!" She made it well known among his coworkers that she did not like him because he was "too fat."

Fellow employees laughed at Loren and chastised him for his appearance. They refused to recognize how well he did his job. Attorneys would whisper and snicker whenever he appeared in court. They would say: "Why is he so fat? He looks horrible! What an embarrassment he is! He sure sweats a lot! He could lose weight if he really wanted to!" They thought he did not hear what they were saying, but Loren heard every hurtful word, each disparaging remark, every jeer and sneer. One day on a visit to a juvenile's home, someone left an anonymous note on Loren's car window: "Clean yourself up, you fat, disgusting, government pig!"

Loren gained his weight over an eight-year period following his mother's death. He cared for his mother in his home during her prolonged illness with cancer, which left her bedridden and blind. Loren was the parent to his mother, and he and his wife cared for her daily physical needs. Her condition deteriorated so much that visiting nurses refused to attend to her.

Ultimately, Loren had no choice but to put her in a nursing home for the last two weeks of her life. This was something that he swore he would never do. She died on his birthday when he had only been on his new job as a probation officer for three days. Deep feelings of guilt and grief drove him to the lowest point in his life. This most important woman—who taught him, nurtured him, provided for him, and loved him unequivocally—was now gone. Loren was devastated.

A deep depression set in. He let his body go. He didn't exercise. He ate everything in sight. He gained so much fat that he grew out of his clothes. He had given up and didn't care how he looked. He refused to allow anyone to take a picture of him and avoided mirrors so that he would not have to look at himself.

Initially I did not fully understand the depth of Loren's grief at his mother's passing. But one evening while talking to him, he revealed a critical detail that brought the relationship between his mother's death and his grief into proper perspective.

What Loren revealed to me that night was that when he was in college, he was involved in a head-on car crash. He was seriously injured and on his arrival at the hospital, the doctors felt there was little that they could do for him. When his mother arrived at the hospital, the doctors told her that they were about to pronounce her son dead.

Loren's mother pleaded with the doctor. "Please don't give up on him," she implored.

The doctor looked into Loren's mother's eyes, went back into the emergency room, and brought Loren back to life. He was in intensive care for three days, in traction for a month. It took him nine months to learn to walk again, and when he graduated—the first person in his family to do so—he hobbled on stage with a cane to get his diploma.

His mother was responsible for his life, but she was now dead; perhaps Loren felt he should be dead, too. He certainly wasn't taking care of himself. It took a small boy to finally pierce this morose defense.

Loren was shuffling around the local grocery store one evening when he was spied by a five-year-old with a flair for the dramatic and the rude. On seeing Loren in the checkout line, the five year-old shouted to his mother in some amazement and with some disgust, "Look, Mommy; look at that big, fat man."

Everybody laughed.

"It was the most humiliating moment of my life," says Loren. "I had been a police officer in great shape, and now I had sunk to this. It made me so angry that I vowed at that moment to fight back. I vowed to lose the weight," remembers Loren.

Goaded by this embarrassment, the psychic landscape began to change. The elements were reconfigured into a healthier picture.

"It took me eight years to realize that I could not and would not give up on myself, and that I had to change or die. Anything less from me would have trivialized what my mother had done to save my life. I made a commitment not to let the memory of my mother down, by getting fit," says Loren.

With his emotional energy now released rather than restrained, Loren threw himself into affirming life by adopting the three D's: Desire, Discipline, and Determination.

Loren's Three-D approach to commitment: Desire, Discipline, and Determination.

Initially his desire manifested itself as a hunger for knowledge. Loren recognized that knowledge is power and set about learning as much as he possibly could about nutrition, weight loss, and fitness. He continues to research these topics on a daily basis.

Loren also developed the discipline of what he calls the "warrior mentality." He knew he was in the battle for his life and had to show up to win the war.

"My heritage is Irish-Canadian, and most of my ancestors were fighters; they had to fight to survive. So I visualize every workout as an act of survival in my war against fat. Whenever I don't feel like working out, I push myself to do it anyway, and these are often the most satisfying sessions," says Loren.

Terrific Tactic

Visualize exercise workouts as a battle against fat, a real act of survival.

Complacency is not a word in Loren Kelly's vocabulary. Loren is determined never to miss a workout. There are no excuses; it's as simple as that. It has reached the point where the workouts are so reinforcing that he does not want to miss them anyway. They give him a sense of inner peace and energy that he has never before experienced.

Never miss a workout. It's an appointment with yourself that you have to keep.

Using his desire, discipline, and determination in combination with a daily food and exercise diary, weekly attendance at meetings, and incredible support from his group, Loren lost seventy-three pounds in eighteen months. He went from a size fifty-two to a size forty. He felt like a different person. He is a different person.

Now he can get restful sleep and breathe on his own without depending on a machine to breath for him. Now he can run up the stairs rather than sit at the bottom of them. Now he can bend over and tie his shoes instead of asking his kids to tie them. Now he can look in the mirror and not feel ashamed. Now he doesn't need asthma medication because he no longer has asthma attacks.

Improved energy leads to better work habits. Administrators could no longer overlook his good work ethics, and Loren was promoted to a supervisory position. His previous supervisor, who had discriminated against him because of his obesity, became discouraged with her position and quit. Loren now supervises and trains probation officers, something he would never have had the self-esteem to do when he weighed over three hundred pounds.

Loren has never been one for deprivation—healthy eating and good workouts are what helped him. He walks twenty-four miles a week on a treadmill and at the local recreation-center walking track. He also uses weight machines for his resistance work. He admits that he has turned his living room into a gym, but for Loren exercise is about living. Living to see his family grow up.

Loren experienced what it was like to struggle to lose weight, and he refused to allow food to control his life. He discovered that no matter how much he weighed he absolutely and positively had the power to change, and no one could take that away from him. He was ultimately accountable for every pound that he had gained and lost. If he was overweight then he was responsible for it. Loren found out what worked for him, put his very heart and soul into it, and worked exceptionally hard at doing well at it.

This once-obese probation officer is now an inspiration to friends and family.

"I think of that grocery store line, and I cry tears for that fat man. And I know he could come back at any time," says Loren.

Wherever you go, go with all your heart. — Confucius

Crossing the Line—Mary Kay Stiles

It doesn't take much to cross the line from passion to obsession, especially when nothing less than identity and self-image is at stake. Mary Kay Stiles describes how her weight concerns turned into an eating disorder. Her story traces her voyage from obsession back to passion.

In college, as a Resident Assistant (RA) on campus, I took seminars and read books to learn about things that could happen to students who are away from home for the first time. Things like depression, drinking and drugs, suicide, date rape. Even eating disorders like bulimia and anorexia nervosa. The thought never occurred to me that some day I might have one of those unfortunate problems.

My best friend since nursery school was bulimic; her teeth were being destroyed by the acid from her stomach. My college roommate began making herself throw up after eating or drinking alcohol. I couldn't understand why either of them would do such a thing to herself. I thought they had everything going for them.

In my first semester of my senior year of college, I went on a clinic diet with my bulimic roommate. She thought this diet would help her overcome her problem and help her lose her unwanted weight. I weighed about 128 pounds. By Christmas I was down to 109 pounds. I admit I looked pretty skinny, but I still thought I could lose more. But it seemed more was never enough. I could always do better, go lower, get thinner.

Once I got into that mindset I hated what I saw when I looked in the mirror. If I didn't like what I saw, how could anyone else? And so began the cycle of yo-yo dieting that lasted about thirteen years. I'd weigh myself two, three times a day, sometimes more. I'd look in the mirror and see every tiny flaw. I'd see my protruding belly, my fat thighs, my big hips. The scale read ninety-three pounds, but that wasn't accurate; it couldn't have been because the mirror didn't lie. Or did it?

My mind was lying to me, not the mirror. Others would tell me I looked great. Or I was too thin. Still others would say I didn't look healthy. But I never listened. What did they know?

My really serious problems with my abnormal mindset and my weight began when I found out I was pregnant with my son, and his father walked out on me after I told him the news. All he could say was, "I think you should have an abortion." We had had problems in our relationship before I discovered I was pregnant.

That's about the same time I decided to start taking over-the-counter appetite suppressants to curb my appetite and help me lose weight. Maybe if I looked different, changed my hairstyle, changed the way I dress, or lost a few pounds, maybe the relationship would miraculously get better? Yeah right. When things are going good in a relationship, you're happy and you like yourself and your appearance. When things take a turn for the worse, your mindset changes and you try to compensate. What if I change? Will he like me again? Will things get better?

No. The relationship was over. Was I an emotional eater or, should I say, an emotional non-eater? Absolutely. I would not eat sometimes unless I absolutely had to. I'd eat with my family to keep up the appearance of being healthy and taking care of myself. I'd eat at a business lunch because my presence at that lunch was expected. But I didn't join my coworkers in the cafeteria or go out to lunch with them when asked because I didn't think I needed to eat. I may have been hungry, but I always told them I wasn't. I stopped carrying money with me so that I wouldn't be tempted to actually buy food.

But when I would decide to carry money with me to work, I'd end up being so hungry I'd eat the worst possible things for me—a pint of

Ben & Jerry's Ice Cream, four servings per container, 210 calories and seventeen grams of fat per serving. I'd feel such a sense of guilt for having eaten it that the cycle would begin again. "You can't eat now for two days." I saw myself as overweight. I was fixated on my weight. *I was obsessed by it.*

I allowed my mind to control me. I didn't eat, not because I wasn't hungry but because I didn't want to gain any weight. I wanted to lose weight and lots of it. My weight totally consumed my every thought. But I never stopped to consider the consequences of my eating habits.

My son was born nine weeks prematurely. I had to help him in every possible way to be just like every other child born at forty weeks gestation; I had to help him "catch up." Part of that meant giving him as many of my immunities as could possibly be transferred through breast milk. When you don't eat you stop lactating. I couldn't nurse him anymore. What had I done to him?

More guilt. A vicious, never-ending cycle. Up, down, happy, sad, calm, angry, sensitive, apathetic. Everything I felt added fuel to my sense of poor self-esteem.

Despite these thoughts, however, it was undeniable that I enjoyed feeling hungry and not giving in to it because it gave me a sense of control that I didn't seem to have in any other area of my life. I liked being in control, even if it was only over myself. I saw my weight go lower and lower on the scale, and this gave me a sense of accomplishment. My body image changed, too. I didn't look the same in the mirror. I thought I still looked too fat but at least not as fat as the day or week before.

This yo-yo cycle eventually caught up with me. I had a gall bladder attack in the middle of the night. I woke up feeling like my lung had collapsed. I couldn't breathe. The EMTs of the ambulance crew were treating me as if I'd had a heart attack. I was scared. Could I have done something like this to myself? Did I bring this on myself by my bizarre eating habits?

My doctor told me he thought I should weigh about 105 pounds. I thought he was out of his mind. I started reading about what causes gall bladder problems. I also started thinking about how I was to blame for my gall bladder attack. I did some research and sought help by calling an eating disorders clinic. I was told by a counselor over the phone that my answers to her questions showed that I had eleven of thirteen signs of anorexia nervosa and I should seek help. I had already taken the first step. I recognized that what I was doing to myself was not good for me.

Just before my gall bladder was taken out, I weighed ninety-three pounds. I was on an almost fat-free diet to prevent another attack. I thought I looked fantastic; everyone else thought I looked sick. Here we go again with my mind playing tricks on me.

I knew that if I didn't change my ways of thinking, I could end up doing irreversible harm to myself. Eventually I settled into a routine at work and at home, and my weight slowly but surely came back. I was slowly learning to become comfortable again with eating all kinds of food after having my gall bladder removed. Before the surgery I was deathly afraid of eating anything with any kind of fat in it for fear I would have another full-blown gall bladder attack. I was also preoccupied with my career. I was making a name for myself in risk management, a field that had been dominated by men. I have established myself there now, currently being the risk manager for a company that has over two hundred locations in fifteen states.

I gradually went from eating once every two days or so to eating normally. I found that my food diary was an essential reality check for me. Obviously I couldn't simply wing it—I had already learnt that my mind would play tricks on me. Everything I ate or drank that contained calories went into this diary. I weighed food portions and counted fat grams and sodium.

When I began to research eating disorders and read more about them, I came to a realization and an understanding of what I was really doing to myself. And quite honestly it scared me. I was a single parent, working a full-time job and raising a child on my own. My son depended upon me for everything. I had an awesome responsibility. I had to get myself together.

Through reading self-help books and weight-loss books, I learned how to accept myself for what I am. I realized that I was not perfect and probably never would be. I still held on to my perfectionist beliefs, but I eased up somewhat on myself. I developed a new philosophy for myself: What you see is what you get. And if you don't like it that's your problem, not mine.

I also came to the realization that I can't live my life to make other people happy. All of this took a great deal of introspection and time to come about. It didn't happen overnight. I had to focus on me for the first time in my life, in a way I had never seen myself before. I started viewing myself not as fat or ugly or not good enough but as someone who is beautiful—whether people told me that or not. I started to see myself as someone who needed help. I never asked for help before— perfectionists don't; they already know everything. I had to learn how to accept compliments. I had to love myself like I'd never loved myself before—unconditionally. I learned strength, conviction, pride, humility, self-confidence. The list is endless.

I opened my eyes to my possibilities instead of to my shortcomings. I wanted to lose weight to feel good about me. I wasn't losing weight anymore for anyone or anything else. That's what changed, too. Those scales at my weekly meeting are the only scales I get on anymore, outside of going to the doctor. They keep me honest and on track.

Terrific Tactic

Weigh only once a week. Anything more is a set-up for disappointment.

I do the things I do now not because I have to or think I should, but because I want to. Maybe it's just a matter of growing up and maturing. I really like who I am and where I am in my life right now. I couldn't have said that with so much certainty in the past. Overall I'm pretty happy being me.

Independence Day—Dennis McGinnis

Here is a story of persistence in the face of adversity from a humble man with a terrific message.

Dennis McGinnis was always very athletic. He started as a fullback on his school football team when he was a freshman. He was a picture of health in the army where, ironically, this gentle man was a demolition expert. When he left the service he was in great shape, filling his six-foot, four-inch frame with 239 pounds.

After the service Dennis drove cement trucks. He did that for twenty years until the company closed down. He had been content driving those cement trucks. He enjoyed it because he met a lot of people, and it kept him physically active. He then became an over-the-road hauler. The job was nowhere near as physical, and four years later he had gained more than a hundred pounds, now weighing 359 pounds.

The new job had dampened Dennis' spirits and his self-esteem. He stopped caring about his appearance, and his wife and daughter didn't bother him about his weight—yet. They knew he wasn't ready.

But by 1993 Dennis was ready, and he entered the TOPS group where his wife had had some success. His reaction to his first meeting was positive.

"I was made to feel so special. I expected to lose weight, and I knew I would get great support," recalls Dennis.

Having finally made the effort to face the demons and change his lifestyle, Dennis threw himself into his weight-loss efforts. He started by eating smaller portions and counting fat intake. Within the first three weeks he had lost fifteen pounds. Dennis was feeling hopeful again.

While driving his truck three weeks into the attempt to change his life, life changed. A young trainee crane operator swung his boom too low and too fast, hitting a load of steel that was on Dennis' trailer. Dennis saw what was happening but was frozen.

"I was just too heavy and out of shape to get out of the way," says Dennis. "All I could see were five or six pieces of building steel falling down on me."

When the dust settled Dennis had a broken femur, broken left knee, broken left and right ankles, and four broken ribs, and two fingers were barely attached to his right hand.

So much for a new start in life. Instead of losing weight and getting back into shape, Dennis was faced with a life of inactivity and despair.

Dennis was in traction for four months, not the six weeks he had originally been told. He was in a wheelchair for nine months. His fingers had been sewed back on, but he hated the idea of being handicapped. He had army buddies who had been paralyzed, and he knew how they suffered—how they lost their freedom to live normal lives. As an active man who loved to play basketball he didn't want to walk with a limp, yet he had no muscle tone in his legs.

His spirits plummeted. Life seemed too cruel.

"When I looked at all the injuries to my legs I thought I would never be able to drive again, much less play sports or be active," recalls Dennis.

It was going to get worse. Two months after the accident his firm filed for bankruptcy, leaving him with no recourse and no insurance. It wasn't just his ribs, ankles, and thighbone that were broken that day, so was his wallet. He couldn't provide income, help his wife, or attend his daughter's functions, let alone attend to her needs.

Dennis survived this period of despondency and deep depression by praying and doing a lot of soul searching. But it was tough. There were tremendous physical problems and huge financial pressure, not to mention a totally uncertain future. Deep down Dennis was not going to let his situation get the better of him. He vowed to use whatever resources at his disposal to survive. Most of those resources were his faith and the faith of other people.

Despite Dennis's refusal to be broken there were occasions when feelings of despair were overwhelming. On one occasion Dennis wheeled his chair to the basement door and opened it. He stayed there, teetering on the edge of the basement stairs, contemplating releasing the brake and letting the chair crash fatally into the basement. His family could collect the life insurance, and he would no longer be a burden to them or himself. He sat there precariously as time slowed down, numb and yet in tremendous pain. Dennis is a Catholic, however, and believes suicide to be wrong. He knew that wasn't the answer. There was a better way of handling the problem.

"I called my wife at work and told her I needed her to come home at once. She came home, and we talked for a long time. Really openly and honestly. Then we prayed together, and I was able to see that I could make it through. Her dad had a favorite saying—'God never gives you more than you can handle'—and she told me we could all manage this together," says Dennis.

After this intimate exchange Dennis vowed to get more involved with his family. He had been aloof from them for far too long. He started eating dinner with his wife and daughter instead of just retreating to his room.

"I was trying very hard not to detach myself from the people who were helping me the most," says Dennis.

Dennis redoubled his already intense efforts to recover physically. He worked very hard in physical therapy and began regaining his strength. After more dedication and endless exercises Dennis was getting the feeling back in his fingers. Eventually he was able to dispense with the wheelchair.

By the time Dennis was back on his feet the inactivity and challenges of the previous eighteen months showed. It wasn't that he had put back the fifteen pounds he had lost just prior to the accident. He also had gained thirty-one pounds and now topped the scales at 390 pounds, or would have if he had chosen to get on the scales.

Still depressed and certainly avoiding the weight issue, Dennis limped along.

Because of his incapacity Dennis had not been able to go anywhere with his daughter for almost two years. Now that he was more mobile he decided he would take his daughter to the movies. It was independence day. Dennis found his inspiration at the movies, although not in the way you might expect.

He was really looking forward to having a special father-daughter outing. He was still depending on a cane so that standing in line for twenty minutes was really painful. He did, though, and eventually he and his daughter, Theresa, made their way to the theater. As Dennis and his daughter walked through the theater, some teenage boys remarked in a very loud voice, "Hope that fat guy doesn't break the seat."

Once in the movies Theresa held her dad's hand. "It doesn't matter, Dad; they're just a couple of jerks."

She was right about the last part of her comment but wrong about the first. It did matter very much. Dennis cried through the whole movie, which, even to this day, he can't remember—not even the title.

"I could have endured abuse for a long time on my own, but now this involved my daughter. It had the biggest impact on my life," says Dennis.

When Dennis got home he took his wife into the bedroom and told her what happened. They cried together for a while. It was independence day.

A week later Sandra, Dennis's wife, saw a newspaper article about a man in a TOPS group in Topeka who had lost sixty-three pounds in ninety days.

"I remember Sandra saying that she thought it was unbelievable that a person could do that well. That made me want to brag, and I said that I could do better than that," says Dennis.

That next weekend Sandra got Dennis to agree to attend an all-you-can-eat buffet at the local church. It certainly turned out to be all he could handle. It wasn't a buffet but a TOPS meeting.

To his credit Dennis did not feel duped by his wife's effort. He took the surprise in his stride.

"I knew I needed it."

Dennis weighed-in at 403 pounds, which was, ironically, a bit of a relief.

"I thought I weighed more, and I was worried about breaking the scales. I remember seeing a long line of people at the church, waiting to weigh-in. I was worried that they would not have a scale that could weigh me. The weight recorder was a small energetic lady named Mary Jo Artzer. She gave me such a warm welcome and told me that she was so happy I had given this group a chance to help. She said, 'Dennis, it doesn't matter if you have a hundred pounds to lose or twenty; always set small goals. You can do it!' After the meeting I thanked Sandra for helping me change my life."

Dennis felt as if his prayers had been answered and his belief in himself vindicated. Once re-involved Dennis again decided to throw himself into his weight-change effort. Having heard about the man who had lost sixty-three pounds in ninety days, he once again rose to the challenge by announcing to the group, "I bet I can beat that."

"Oh sure!" they all replied.

Mary Jo's suggestion to set small, manageable goals was valuable advice. Dennis decided he was going to focus on losing just ten pounds at a time.

Hope had returned.

"I have a chance for another life."

In the first week he lost fifteen and a half pounds. In ninety days he had lost sixty-seven pounds, winning his challenge with the group. By the end of the year, from the middle of July, Dennis lost over eighty-seven pounds. It was after that he was able to walk without a cane. Remarkably Dennis had lost the weight without being able to do any exercise!

He had managed this by severely cutting back on his red-meat intake and replacing it with turkey and chicken. He once again reduced his portions and added lots of fruits and vegetables. Importantly, Sandra and Theresa ate the same foods as Dennis, didn't keep any tempting foods around the house, and kept praising and encouraging him.

Throwing his cane away meant getting back to exercise. On the first day he drove himself to the mall and walked for the first time in nearly two years. He walked half a mile and was laid up in bed for the next three days as a result. The following week he did the same thing, and this time he was bedridden for only two days. Progress.

It took Dennis about a month to walk that distance without too many subsequent problems. Others started to join him in his mall walking. Helen German had started at TOPS the same day as Dennis, and soon she was walking with him in the mall. Before long others had joined so that there was a regular group walking the mall.

"I really appreciated them walking with me because I definitely needed moral support to keep me motivated," says Dennis.

Within a few months Dennis added an exercise bike to his routine. In that year, he lost another sixty-two pounds. Along the way, he hit several plateaus, but Dennis just kept going, refusing to be deflected by weeks of no weight loss. He had a rule that helped him.

"Once off, never back on," he vowed.

Dennis is an inspiration to his group and in his area. So is his wife, who herself lost seventy-two pounds when she joined TOPS. Together Dennis and Sandra are the first husband-wife area captains in Kansas.

Dennis is eternally grateful to those who helped him turn his life around. He travels the state, giving motivational talks—a helpful, kind man who, with dedication and commitment, has turned despair into joy.

Dennis still walks the malls, and sometimes you can see him with Helen German, who lost sixty-three pounds the year he lost eighty-seven.

Two months ago Mary Jo Artzer, the person who had weighed Dennis when he re-entered TOPS, saw him in the mall. She gave Dennis a big hug, a small butterfly charm, and a card that simply said, "Friends Forever." Last week Dennis learned that Mary Jo had passed away.

Dennis has the same passion for life as Mary Jo did. His commitment and drive have taken him back from the precipice and will serve him well, no matter what the future brings.

It's not that I am so smart, it's just that I stay with problems longer. – Albert Einstein

Nursing School—Patsy Casteen

A man has got to do what a man has got to do. So does a woman. Here is a story of tremendous commitment in life, as well as weight loss.

When Patsy Casteen's husband was disabled ten years ago with a serious back injury, she knew she had to step up to the plate. She had been stepping up and sitting down in front of food plates for some time, and her waistline showed it. Here, however, was a different sort of challenge. Her family's welfare depended on it.

Patsy had a degree in cosmetology, but the local economy would not support another such venture; in any event Patsy now needed the security of a reliable, regular income. So she chose to pursue a nursing career. Unfortunately she wasn't qualified. She determined, however, that lack of credentials was no reason to be deflected from this particular goal.

Lacking some fundamental courses, Patsy enrolled in a local college and began taking core classes that would be required for her nursing career. It had been a long time since she had been in an academic environment and twenty-two years since she had graduated from high school. Patsy was determined, however, to overcome any problems that might occur as a result of being a mature student who had been out of the studying business for two decades. Hard work would make up for whatever else she might lack, she thought.

It wasn't studying that presented the only problem, though. Patsy also had to earn some money so that the family could live. She took a job working the night shift, eleven at night to seven in the morning, doing clerical work in an orthopedic department. That job unfortunately couldn't meet all the bills, so that when Patsy got off work she went to her second job as a school bus driver. When that job was complete she headed over to the school cafeteria where she spent several hours collecting lunch money. After that she could finally go home— and take care of her disabled husband and three adolescents before getting a few hours of sleep before heading out to school.

Patsy's punishing program persisted for three years. Once she had passed the core material, she was enrolled in nursing school.

"I had to take it hour by hour, sometimes even less than that," says Patsy. "All I would do is eat, sleep, work, and cry," she recalls.

There was time for crying but certainly not for eating healthily. Many meals were eaten on the run, and her stress levels were higher than the cholesterol content of the junk food she was eating. Exercise consisted of physically getting from her night job to her day job to afternoon classes.

Patsy recalls how she fought the incredible stress brought about by her situation. She had received a card on which was written, "Negative-Free Zone." Patsy framed the saying and hung it in her room. Whenever she was getting depressed, when doubts crept in, when she wondered whether she would ever graduate, when she wondered whether it would be all worth it, she went into that room, looked at that framed saying, and determined to chase all negativity away.

Patsy was progressing positively. In fact she had one class left to complete before graduating from nursing school. The end was near. There were further distractions as she now had a grandchild at home. Then she failed her very last nursing course. The stress and demands had finally caught up with her. Moreover the nursing school rules didn't allow students to retake the course for nine months after they had failed it.

Nine more months to sit out. Nine more months before she could get one regular steady job rather than a night job, a day job, and attend school. So Patsy did what she always did: she gritted her teeth and made the best of a difficult situation.

When she returned to school to finish her training she connected with two classmates, and they studied together. Previously Patsy had been studying alone; there simply was not enough time to add study time with classmates into her already overwhelming schedule. Now with the end in sight, helpful camaraderie, and her typical determination, Patsy was able to put in the work required to pass. She didn't just pass; she passed with flying colors.

Shortly after graduating from college she took a full-time nursing position at a nearby hospital. It took a while to get acclimated to a new career and work situation, but Patsy made the adjustment. However, there was a new challenge just around the corner.

Through this ordeal of retraining herself, Patsy simply had neither the time nor the attention to make weight loss a priority. Her weight had ballooned to 260 pounds. On a flight to England to visit one of her daughters, her legs swelled badly, and she constantly had to leave her seat, drawing disgusted glances and comments from fellow passengers. She stood for five hours of the nine-hour flight.

Part of the problem was that Patsy was on the verge of congestive heart failure. She had been throwing her heart into everything she did so that it's no wonder it was beginning to wear out. One evening she had to be rushed to the hospital where she admits, "I thought I was going to die."

With her life now in better order because of her work and financial situation and God giving her warning signs, Patsy turned her attention to losing weight. Characteristically, Patsy threw herself into her weight loss. She joined a small group and attended regularly. She set very short-term goals for herself. Previously it had been one hour at a time; now it was literally a quarter pound at a time. She used her group, as well as Internet buddies, for support when she felt her resolve slipping. She set a variety of tasks that would distract her if she was feeling hungry or tempted. One of these was scrapbooking. Looking at pictures of family and friends seemed to get her grounded again in the important things in life. Exercise, too, became a part of Patsy's life. She walked several miles almost every day. And she spent a lot of time in the "Negative-Free Zone."

Terrific Tactic

Create a negative-free zone—a place of peace where you check all troubles, worries, and stress at the door.

It has been three years now since Patsy became a nurse and two since she lost the 110 pounds that burdened her frame. Looking back on the struggles of the past few years, Patsy frankly admits, "I don't know how I did it."

Patsy is now the leader of her group and always looking for new programs or stories to inspire the many new members she has helped to recruit. She doesn't have to look very far.

Rankin's Reminders

Making Priorities; Getting Passionate

Make the decision. Anything is possible once you have decided to do it.

Go public. Tell as many people as possible about your goals.

Define your goals. Be specific. Make goals tangible, behavioral targets (e.g., I'm not going to eat more than thirty grams of fat a day) rather than vague ideas (e.g., I'm going to lose ten pounds).

Write a contract. Write a contract that specifies what behaviors you are going to change.

Start with one behavior. Begin by focusing on one specific behavior and mastering it. For example, walk thirty minutes a day or eliminate dessert.

Make it a priority. Write exercise times down in your diary, and keep them as sacred appointments. Whatever else happens, ensure you meet your goal for the day.

Stay connected to your motivation. Remember the pain that made you want to lose weight in the first place.

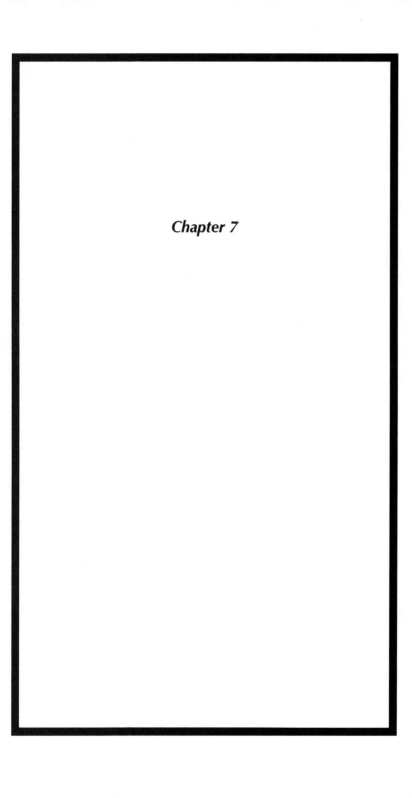

Chapter 7

The Connection of Souls

Help others to help yourself

A friend is someone who knows the song in your heart and can sing it back to you when you have forgotten the words. – Anonymous

---

The stories in this book are a testament to the concept that personal support and a close connection with at least one other human being are essential for serious weight loss and lifestyle change. An open, real, supportive, and loving relationship provides many tools for the weight struggle: information, a balanced perspective, encouragement, an opportunity to express feelings, a reality check on behavior, and a model for success — to name but a few.

Intimacy, not to be confused with just physical intimacy, is a meaningful, interpersonal connection. It is the direct one-to-one connection stripped away of all pretense and defense. For so many weight is a barrier to such a connection. Extra pounds are a shell in which to hide and, by and large, the strategy works. A physical shell isn't really needed if you have a psychological one, but because the body is the outward manifestation of the mind, physical walls and psychological walls tend to occur together. Breaking down these walls is the key to successful lifestyle change.

This book is filled with stories of people who were coerced, encouraged, motivated, supported, and loved enough so that they could escape unhealthy habits and reclaim their lives. If pain and hurt lead to weight gain, love and friendship can lead to weight loss.

If pain and hurt lead to weight gain, love and friendship can lead to weight loss.

Intimacy, love, and friendship all begin with trust. Trust is not just about keeping secrets and respecting confidence. *Trust comes at the moment you know that your deepest feelings, thoughts, and desires will be unconditionally respected.* Friends may not always agree with you or even understand you, but they will always respect your right to think and feel the way you do.

Far too many people are raised in environments where trust does not exist, where they are made to doubt the validity of their feelings, and where they are made to feel ashamed of their anger. Many people have little or no experience with validation or recognition. The only way to escape from that prison is to experience the freedom that true intimacy brings. If you haven't had much success with trust, however, it is difficult to initiate the interaction that leads to it. Entering a supportive group environment is a good way to break free from isolation. In such a group time can be spent initially observing interactions and getting comfortable with the environment without risking too much personal involvement and vulnerability. Once a comfort level is reached, sharing and trusting can really begin.

Excess weight cannot only be a general barrier but also a wall erected as a defense in a specific relationship. If that specific relationship is a major one—for example, with a spouse—defensiveness can be all-encompassing. It can consume the individual and come to affect all aspects of life, permeating into all other relationships. You might be fat because you are angry with your husband, but that excess weight and the consequent frustration is there for everyone to see.

As a marriage therapist I know that many couples live in an intimacy blackout. They don't trust each other, rarely share innermost feelings, and then wonder why their sex lives are so bad. Viagra is no substitute for trust. Often this intimacy void is not a function of anger or resentment but simply the reluctance or inability to expose thoughts, feelings, and desires. That reluctance comes from fear of rejection, ridicule, or simply not being taken seriously. Unconditional acceptance can overcome this reticence and be incredibly empowering. Once a foundation of trust is laid, all manner of personal transformations and miracles can occur. Simply opening up to another person has tremendously therapeutic properties.

Enormous psychic energy is expended in keeping strong emotions trapped in the unconscious and thus the body. It is an old axiom that depression is anger "turned inward." When anger is unexpressed, energy is required to keep the lid on it. This is tremendously draining, and soon the person burdened by this situation is exhausted. Depression is an energy problem more than anything else so that whenever strong emotions remain trapped, mood disturbance and depression are likely to occur. Venting the emotion, simply by talking to another person, releases the pressure and can restore an amazing amount of energy.

A mutually trusting relationship requires accountability, too. If I make a commitment to report my weight to another person on a weekly basis, I now have to be accountable to that person *and to me*. I can't so easily deceive myself, make excuses, or simply wait until I feel I'm being successful to get back on the scales.

Honesty is a requisite of a meaningful conversation. When discussing personal issues in a real, connected conversation, two important things happen. First you hear yourself. Hearing thoughts and feelings expressed out loud is powerful. In the absence of a confidante, our innermost and deepest thoughts simply rattle around unexpressed in our heads where it is much easier for them to be distorted, forgotten, or ignored. Once feelings are expressed, however, they are born into the world and have an existence that cannot be denied. So a second consequence of a real discussion is honesty. Sharing feelings makes them real. You cannot run or hide from them.

Openly expressing thoughts also makes them subject to evaluation. This is why open expression is often not forthcoming, but that is precisely why it should be. Human beings are psychological animals, not logical ones. It is important for us to subject our thoughts to a reality check.

It's much easier solving other people's problems because those issues can be seen without the filters of the ego. True friends are able to offer nonjudgmental reality checks. Such "anchoring" is the cornerstone of support.

When you make real contact with another person you are helping two people. Extending oneself is valuable because it not only has the power to motivate others, but it also reinforces your own beliefs. There's nothing like public commitment to reinforce commitment, as demonstrated in the chapter on Priority and Passion. Many people featured in this book find their motivational speaking an important part of their own ability to maintain weight loss and a healthy lifestyle.

In my book, *Power Talk: The Art of Effective Communication*, I make the point that communication is a spiritual exercise because truly listening and trying to understand another involves temporarily stepping outside personal boundaries. Recognizing there is something greater than your own ego is the essence of spirituality. Venturing outside psychological defenses is an important part of venturing beyond physical defenses.

Finding people whom you can trust and with whom you can make the connection is no easy feat. A positive group is the ideal place to start because it affords some safety and an environment to initially observe. In a group there will be like-minded people, and the chances are that there will be someone with whom you can relate. Moreover, social psychological research shows that identification is greatly enhanced when people share at least one common goal.

Intimacy does not necessarily have to come from a group, however. There are people all around who might fulfill the role of trusted confidante. They could be spouses, siblings, family members, coworkers, or friends. In this chapter I have chosen examples from each of these areas.

At the time of need, the value of support is not so much in convincing people to make better food choices or avoid temptation but to give them a real connection—the most important source of comfort there is.

Everybody can be great because anybody can serve. You don't have to have a college degree to serve. You don't have to make your subject and verb agree to serve. You only need a heart full of grace. A soul generated by love. – Martin Luther King

A Mountain to Climb—Gary Wellington

Gary Wellington, a man who quite literally climbed a mountain, needed the love and support of his wife to recover from a near fatal pulmonary embolism.

Gary and Carlene Wellington have been married nearly forty years. Four decades of typical ups and downs. Today they are closer than ever.

For many years their marriage followed a typical path. Gary was a hard-drinking, hard-working guy, a metaphorical fighter who had let his weight balloon so that even his size sixty pants could be a little tight. He liked the outdoors, especially hunting and fishing, but his weight had prevented him from realizing his dream of climbing nearby Mt. Rainier. Carlene was the caretaking mother who put up with a lot. Their marriage drifted along on the sea of daily tasks and chores. They talked but rarely communicated.

All that changed one week in the spring of 1990. Gary's poor eating, lack of exercise, and obesity made him a poor health risk. After a week of not feeling well, a trip from the family room to his bedroom—a climb of thirty-nine stairs—left him faint and gasping for breath. Carlene was concerned and suggested that he take an aspirin, go to bed, and see a doctor in the morning. The next day Gary was no better, but he dismissed the discomfort with characteristic stubbornness. A friend, Chris, came by later that evening and walked outside with Gary to help him feed a few cattle. They had just about reached the barn when Gary found himself gasping for breath. He felt the strength drain from him, and he told Chris that he was "going down." Chris ran back to the house and hollered for Carlene to call 911. She thought he was joking, but when she saw the anxiety in his face she knew that this was no joke.

Two ambulances were on the scene within a few minutes.

Gary doesn't remember much about the trip to the hospital. The paramedics were trying desperately to keep him alive. Gary does recall what happened when he reached the hospital, however.

Lying on the gurney, drugged and panicked, Gary heard the ER doctor talking with Carlene. "There's a real good chance that he's not going to make it through the night," said Dr. Blackburn.

Gary was scared to death. Not that he needed to get any closer to mortality; that was already on his shoulder and spreading fast. Gripped in the fear of his impending demise, Gary took one moment at a time, seconds at a time. To ensure that he wasn't going to die, Gary kept one eye open all the time—or tried to. Whenever he would drift out of consciousness, his waking was a cause of incredible relief.

"I'm still here," he thought a hundred times during those first few agonizing hours. Against the odds, Gary made it through the night. The next morning Gary was barely able to speak to Carlene directly.

"I'm sorry," were the first words he said to his wife. Sorry he had denied his problem. Sorry he had made half-hearted attempts to lose weight. Sorry he hadn't listened to Carlene. Sorry that he had put her in that position. Sorry that he didn't know whether he was going to live.

Whether he was going to live was a matter of conjecture. Gary was not afraid to die. He had a good relationship with God, but he wanted a longer one with Carlene. Gary looked at his wife and could see the determination and love in her eyes. He hadn't seen that for a while. He hadn't been looking.

"We got you through last night, but there is still a long way to go, buddy," said Dr. Blackburn when he visited.

Not just a long way—a veritable mountain to climb.

Climbing a mountain requires taking one step at a time. At least now, one day after, those steps were measured in hours rather than seconds. Hours turned into days. Gary spent nine days in the hospital. During that time he and Carlene talked liked they hadn't before.

If Gary had seen his life flash before his eyes like a movie, he would have seen that Carlene was the central character, the best supporting actress. Gary had not been forced to sit through this movie before. Carlene, too, coming so close to losing her male lead, was seeing the man with whom she had fallen in love.

Together they vowed to change their lives. Right now that meant Gary following the doctor's instructions to the letter and preparing for a different life. Carlene's commitment to a new life began immediately. By the time Gary was released from the hospital, Carlene had already set up a bedroom downstairs for him. She had completely revamped her cooking and took full charge of all meals. She carefully measured out portions and completely eliminated any junk food. And she got them both involved in TOPS.

Terrific Tactic

Completely eliminate junk food. If simply passing by the place is tempting, change your route.

Dr. Blackburn was also pushing Gary. He demanded a weight loss of at least a pound a week and told Gary he could forget any hunting trips until he improved his fitness. Gary pushed the envelope. At first he could barely walk a hundred feet but within a month was regularly walking five miles a day and occasionally ten.

With Carlene's love and care, his doctor's advice, and the encouragement of his TOPS friends, Gary lost sixty pounds in five months. He never missed any meetings and was driven by his accountability to the group and especially to Carlene.

"If I had to do it by myself I couldn't have done it," says Gary of his wife's efforts.

They changed their lifestyle, learning new habits together. This togetherness was important and was one of the many things that they now openly shared. Like the fears, their deepest feelings, working together, learning about foods, and learning to talk at the same level.

Terrific Tactic

Sharing thoughts and feelings about food with family members helps them understand what you are going through and thus makes it more likely that they will be supportive.

Within a year Gary had reached his goal by losing ninety-five pounds. Carlene had lost sixty-one pounds. They had helped each other become fitter and stronger, individually and collectively. They participated together in TOPS meetings and events.

One of the TOPS events was a ten-mile walk. It was during preparation for that event that Gary half jokingly mentioned the idea of climbing Mt. Rainier. Carlene wasn't too excited about the idea but others were, and before he knew it Gary was seriously considering the pursuit of his life's dream.

Gary began practicing on the lower elevations of the mountain. On one of his practice runs he met an employee of KING-TV, a large network affiliate in Seattle. Before he knew it Gary was going to be taking a camera with him to record his journey. Instead of having a cameraman from the TV station accompany him, Gary had his son, Gordon, accompany him on the fulfillment of this life goal.

After training for several months the day finally arrived. Reaching the high-elevation camp at ten thousand feet presented few problems for Gary. After preparing themselves for the big climb, Gary and his son set out for the top. They were carrying not only a camera but also a CB radio, cell phone, batteries, and other communications equipment that would keep them in touch not just with KING-TV but also with radio stations that had picked up the story, as well as his closest TOPS friends and, of course, Carlene.

It normally takes six hours to reach the summit at 14,410 feet. As the climb progresses it gets harder and harder, steeper, and it becomes more difficult to breathe. Gary "hit the wall."

"Every step became a tremendous chore. My mind wanted my body to move, but my body couldn't respond," recalls Gary.

Every few paces Gary had to stop to regroup and gather his mental strength. It was entirely mental now. His body was exhausted. He kept talking to himself.

"I can do this."

"You cannot fail."

"You made the commitment."

"The only person left to do this is yourself."

Slowly—painfully and slowly—Gary made his way to the top.

"The only person left to do this is yourself."

When he reached the summit Gary was excited and exhilarated. He started to breathe easier and feel stronger. He also knew, however, that he had to stay focused.

The descent of any mountain climb takes a lot of careful steps. Exhaustion and excitement follow a stressful ascent. With the cold and winds constantly blowing up to thirty miles an hour, Gary knew this was no time to lose focus. *He knew that there are as many accidents on the way down as there are on the way up.*

Gary did not have an accident on the way down. He and his son made it safely to base camp at ten thousand feet and decided to rest the night. The following day they traveled the remaining three miles to the parking lot at five thousand feet. Carlene and their closest TOPS friends were there to greet Gary and his son.

Seeing Gary come down the mountain and enter the camp, Carlene was in tears. She had been apprehensive about the climb, but now she was so proud. Gary, who characteristically did not like any of the fuss made about his effort, walked directly up to Carlene and embraced her. It wasn't just that he had made it. They had made it.

In his motivating speeches Gary draws the parallel between climbing a mountain and losing weight—one step at a time; keep focused; there is as much danger on the way down as there is on the way up. And he also knows that behind every successful mountain climber, there is a dream weaver that makes it all possible.

"There is as much danger on the way down as there is on the way up."

A Friend Indeed—Sharon Nichol

Sharon Nichol found her support in a valued friend and coworker who proved to be an inspiration and a huge motivating force. This is her story.

I have been overweight most of my life, but my first memory of concern was when I was twelve. The kids at school would tease me. I had one girlfriend, and she was overweight, too. The others would call us, "the fat twins." I would come home from school so upset.

My mother would give me a hug and say, "Don't worry; it's just baby fat. You'll grow out of it."

I was the youngest of five children by seven years, so I was the baby and, frankly, spoiled rotten.

My mother contracted scarlet fever as a child, which created some hearing problems. When she was eighteen she suffered a head trauma when playing basketball and lost all of her hearing. My father was born deaf. They overcompensated for these problems by indulging me somewhat, especially with food. If they were ashamed or embarrassed about their conditions, I certainly wasn't. I loved them, and I was proud for all that they achieved despite their handicaps.

In adolescence I did use their hearing problems to my advantage, sometimes sneaking out, thinking—wrongly—that they couldn't hear. My mother was right about a lot of things, including the fact that I would grow out of my "baby fat." By the time I was fourteen I had grown two inches taller and trimmed down to a size ten naturally. From then on I would gain ten pounds in the winter and lose it again in the summer. I didn't realize at the time that all of the summer activities like swimming and walking were really exercise in disguise.

I was what is lovingly called a "free spirit," which really meant that I was willful, independent, and didn't take too kindly to instruction or advice. Hardly surprising then that I dropped out of high school and was married to Mike by the time I was eighteen.

When I got married I wore a size twelve wedding dress. A year later I got pregnant with my first daughter and actually lost weight because I was sick all the time. It was not just motherhood that was making me sick. When I was five months pregnant my mother and sister were killed in a car accident. I was angry, confused, excited about being pregnant, and frightened of having a baby without my mother and sister there to help me.

By the time I had my second and then third daughter, however, I was wearing a size sixteen. Up until this point I had not really ever tried to lose weight, but now the weight was making me uncomfortable.

I started by severely restricting my diet, but every few days I would pig out because I was starving. Then I was on a modified Slim Fast program. I would stay on the Slim Fast during the day and reward myself with candy at night. Before long I put back the few pounds that I lost initially and just gave up. Finally I got to the point where I didn't care what I looked like. As long as I avoided mirrors and cameras and didn't have to see the real me, I thought I could live with it.

This denial went on for ten years until 1996 when I weighed approximately two hundred pounds. Now I was wearing a size twenty. Mike, who had been incredibly supportive, stopped paying attention to me and was telling me that he missed the way we used to be. I was hurt, but we worked hard on our communication to resolve the problem. But even that didn't motivate me to lose weight, even though I was breathless walking up stairs and was still avoiding seeing my reflection. Deep down I was hiding.

My husband and I had smoked since we were teenagers, but it was now giving us some problems. Mike, in particular, was suffering with asthma. I honestly did not want to quit, but I wanted to support his efforts. I used some nicotine patches and spent three solid days reading up in my bedroom (where I never smoked).[1] So we successfully quit smoking. Mike's asthma got better, and I gained another fifty pounds. The doctor was more concerned about my smoking than weight, and I didn't realize that the nicotine was elevating my metabolism.[2]

Now at nearly 250 pounds I really started to suffer. I was tired all the time. I was frequently breathless. And the heavier I got the more withdrawn I became. I was almost reclusive at this point. I still didn't like my reflection and would barely look in the mirror at my face. One day when I did, I saw that my eyelid was drooping. After numerous visits to the doctor I was diagnosed with a neuromuscular disease called Myasthenia Gravis. I was told that this was not weight related, so I continued to eat the same way I always had, including one pound bags of M&M's for dessert. It's no wonder I started having acid reflux, often waking up in the middle of the night, choking. Back to the doctor, who suggested losing a few pounds and cutting out the nighttime snacks.

I don't know why this is what finally motivated me to do something about my weight. I wasn't feeling afraid, and I didn't feel threatened or pushed. Perhaps that's why I responded. Perhaps that strong-willed side of me was determined not to give in until then. It didn't feel like giving in—just taking the advice of a respected professional.

Not that the decision was easy. I really wasn't sure that I wanted to change my habits or give up the food that I loved. But I started to think about my daughters, and I realized that I wanted to see them grow up. I wanted to grow old with my best friend, Mike.

A colleague, Debbee Sereduck[3], had been going to TOPS and was being very successful. She invited me to the July 4 picnic where I weighed-in at a shade under 250 pounds and promptly left in shock and dismay. I kept my weight a secret and, frankly, wasn't very excited about the prospect of going back.

But Debbee encouraged me to stick with it. She told me that if she could do it, I could, too. She was a constant reminder of what was possible. She had been considerably heavier than I was and had lost a tremendous amount of weight. She also encouraged me in just the right way. If it hadn't been for Debbee's inspiration and support, I'm not sure I would have kept going. Reluctantly I went back to the group.

The more I went, the more support I got, not just from Debbee but from others, too. They made me feel good about myself and understood what I was going through.

I started out eating lots of salads, watched my portions, and drank lots of water. I lost over sixteen pounds in four weeks and thought this is going to be sooooo easy! The next week I weighed, I had gained a little weight. I was so mad! I think that's when I really threw myself into the program. At last I was making my willfulness work for me rather than against me!

If you're angry enough you can give up anything.

I redoubled my efforts. I started counting fat grams, allowing myself thirty daily. I would eat three low-fat meals a day and feel full. I followed my physician's advice and ate nothing after 6 P.M. This really helped with the acid reflux. I made it my business to learn as much as I could about nutrition, food labels, and the like. And all the time Debbee was there encouraging me, along with the other TOPS members.

Terrific Tactic

Don't eat anything after the early evening hours. This allows for proper digestion and better sleep and can eliminate high-calorie nighttime snacks.

Within a couple of weeks I started to exercise—or tried to. My husband is so supportive; he'd walk with me anytime. The first time we went out we had only gone one block before my back hurt badly. I didn't think I was going to make it home. *But I refused to be beaten.*

I started some water-aerobics classes, which were great because I love the water. Gradually I got stronger and was exercising whenever I got the chance. Before long I was doing it three times a week. Now I do it every day.

Soon I was making my weight-loss effort a priority. I put in an enormous amount of effort and refused to be sidetracked by anything or anyone. My program was constantly on my mind, and I would do whatever was necessary to stick with it. Of course, it helped having a supportive husband and three proud kids. And a great friend in Debbee.

The weight rolled off at a fairly consistent eight pounds a month. Within fifteen months I had lost the hundred pounds that my doctor set as a goal. At that point I was down to a size twelve. While learning to maintain I lost another twelve pounds and am now a size eight.

There have been other influences outside my family that have been enormously helpful. In the past I may not have been so receptive to others, choosing instead to be "independent." But without Debbee's help I probably would not have gone to TOPS in the first place, may not have gone back after the first "meeting," and would not have had the wonderful support of a friend, colleague, and walking partner who is truly an inspiration. She inspired me, and I added the determination, commitment, and passion to make it work.

Another of my TOPS pals who helped me was Kathy. Debbee had lost most of her weight by the time I was losing mine, but Kathy had not. She and I enjoyed a healthy, friendly competition that kept us both focused on our goals. Kathy has lost eighty-five pounds to date and is getting ever closer to her goal.

Terrific Tactic

Finding someone with whom you can indulge in "friendly" competition can be motivating. Remember, though, that weight loss is not a competition with another person, but one with yourself.

When I first started losing weight I was not a very spiritual person. As I have lost my weight, however, my faith has increased tremendously. It's almost as if I've opened myself up to let others in and help me.

Today we are a much healthier family. My oldest daughter has lost the thirty pounds she needed to lose, and we all eat much more healthily. Mike has lost thirty pounds, too, and exercises on a regular basis. We are far more active and watch far less television. And my Myasthenia is in remission.

I have learned that you have to be focused and passionate about your efforts. Find support, keep a food chart, and exercise every day. Inspire and be inspired!

It is one of the most beautiful compensations in life that no man can sincerely try to help another without helping himself. – Ralph Waldo Emerson

Love and Fat Cells—Susan Burkholder

Susan Burkholder describes the relationship between intimacy, feeling loved, and weight. Susan's story describes the stages that got her to a healthy place: eliminating dependency, improving self-esteem, making better choices, then losing weight.

When I look back on the snapshots of my life I realize how much of the fluctuation in my weight was tied up with feeling loved or unloved.

In high school I would have been just "chunky," but that was okay—the homecoming queen was chunky, too. I had a steady guy and no problem with getting dates. In fact I was fairly secure in my emotions as I headed off to nurses' training where I learned all about nutrition, hating every minute of the class. The carbohydrate menu would have fattened pigs. I gained weight but not to fear—diet pills were given through the health services in our residence. The pounds of potatoes were shed, and a wonderful 117-pound body emerged. Actually the weight loss was only about fifteen pounds, but it was perfect for finding a mate and wearing the white, long gown to walk down the aisle. LOVED.

Just after the first child three years later, I was dubbed fat by the love of my life. He offered me a whole new wardrobe, money, and just about anything to lose weight. He was the least of my motivators, but skiing was a motivator. Each fall I would work out and train diligently to be prepared for the slopes. I would use many diet books, buying each new one to help me look beautiful. Dieting was a way of life, even if not completely successful.

Through my second pregnancy I played tennis and swam daily in the summer months. I came home from the hospital and was in my cut-off denims within the week. I didn't look fat and have the pictures to prove that I wasn't, but mentally I thought I was.

No, I wasn't fat—just not up to my husband's standards. But then his lovers set the standards, not my figure. My weight gain wasn't huge, but he didn't love me anymore.

There is nothing like a divorce, death, or affair to pull in the waistline. Mine was an affair. Much more emotional than physical, but I shed those extra pounds without a thought to diet. I also was a compulsive eater with the chocolate bars hidden in the drawer under the dishtowels. I could sneak one of those little things and have it down without being caught by children or husband. It wasn't the chocolate that hurt me but the habit—or, better word—addiction. UNLOVED.

Once, after the divorce, my children brought home a sheet cake left over from Daddy's birthday party, which he had given one of them. I ate most of the sheet cake, trying to soothe the hurt. VERY UNLOVED.

I stayed shapely for many years with just little ups and downs. When I fell in love with a man my weight stayed under control, my emotional eating stayed hidden, and sometimes I could even give up smoking, which I did many times. Love filled the bill.

Some crisis times gave way to gaining. For example, moving to another area always put on the pounds. Usually it involved much energy with three children. My first year back in my hometown the scales went to a size fifteen for a time, but careful eating and becoming readjusted helped bring it down. Of course, I met another man, and that scooted it down as well.

Before he and I got married, I was skinny, happy, jogging—and closet eating. He lived out of town, so I was free from his careful eyes most of the time. I even quit smoking on the weekends when we were together. Then we married. Not only had I married another man who didn't have sex at home, he was also even more abusive about calling me fat. Just a wee bit smarter toward the end of the marriage, I noticed he would complain about me not exercising enough; yet it was me climbing out of bed at 5:30 A.M. to hit the gym before work as he lay sleeping. UNLOVED AND UNHAPPY.

The entire marriage was doomed and very unhealthy. I could never please him, so I didn't and gained weight. Lots of it. Our time together was a roller-coaster ride, and I was totally out of control with eating and living. UNLOVED AND EMOTIONALLY FAT.

As I look back, we were both pickers and tried to hide that from each other by eating sweets—not at the table but walking away from each other or when not together. My afternoon at work could consist of two chocolate bars, depending on the stress involved in the day. Sometimes I would cover up the eating by purchasing enough chocolate to go around. Of course, my stash was hidden in the bottom left drawer of my desk. I don't hide food anymore, but at the time I did. Pounds came on and on; dress sizes went up.

Terrific Tactic

Don't hide food. If you're going to eat, don't be ashamed of it. If you are ashamed, perhaps you shouldn't be eating.

This divorce led to three years of counseling. It wasn't all about the marriage but also the realization that for years I had listened to men tell me how I had to look, what size dress I had to wear—all in the name of love. Being in abusive relationships was my norm. Time to change that. My counselor and I worked on my growing up mentally and taking control of my life.

Eating wasn't such a big deal anymore. I was alone, loving it, and I had a male friend who thought I was perfect. He was pretty hefty, but my weight remained stable and under control, even though I wasn't thin.

Fast forward to my late forties, and it's time for a hysterectomy. I felt very empty in my lower abdomen. It was time for hormonal therapy. No one warned me that Premarin puts inches onto the waist. Just the area I'd had trouble with all my life. Not only did the weight come on, but also I was so happy with the hormones, I didn't care. That was a good, ten solid not-going-to-go-away pounds. Anyone for a size sixteen?

Finally I loved myself, even with the extra weight. Oh, I tried diets and lost some, then regained, but no one was telling me how to look or feel and I was okay. LOVED MYSELF.

At the age of forty-nine I moved to Colorado for a job. It had always been a dream to live in Colorado and ski, the greatest passion of my life. The children, now grown, wished me well and sent me down the highway. A new experience just in time to meet my fiftieth birthday. In Colorado my weight didn't fluctuate much, but I was overweight. I tried dieting with Weight Watchers and failed a few times. I had many stressors that caused me to eat more, but I was still okay with me.

Then I met my third husband, stopped smoking, and gained twelve pounds. I became a snowbird, walked daily, and was healthy even with the weight. His perception of me as beautiful, even with the weight, helped me to be happy and heavy. He never hounded me about weight and encouraged me along the way. We made a major lifestyle change from alternating between Colorado and the motor home, traveling to a permanent home in Arizona.

Upon arrival in Arizona, I was finally ready to take weight loss seriously and joined a new group. It has been two years without a cigarette, the twenty pounds is coming off, and I am following the plan. We started a new smaller group in our area. The new group, the new year, and the new me are coming along fine. The weight loss isn't great yet, but the trophy for best loser is on our mantle. My husband woke me this week by lovingly saying: "Good morning loser!"

Weight loss for me has in the past meant being loved or unloved with many shades of these emotions in between. Stress has played a big part as well, but hopefully I am on the right track without any labels— it is just time to get it off, and my support system will help me do it.

I Don't Know—Peggy Malecha

Peggy Malecha's piece epitomizes what sharing is about and how making contact can save lives.

It was just the two of us on that chilly evening, sitting in a small corner of a church, somewhere in the Midwest. I sat there, listening very hard, concentrating — really concentrating — on what she had to say. As I focused every ounce of my energy on the details that were spewing out of her mouth, I lost my self-awareness, totally absorbed in her.

She was just twenty-one. Attractive, bright, and hopelessly out of control. She told me about the uncontrollable binges that went on for days. She confessed to me about the endless doses of laxatives she took by the fistful. She raged about the constant criticism from and rejection by her parents. She cried bitterly about her perfectly thin twin. She agonized relentlessly about her guilt and her shame. She described how she had hidden vomit under her bed to escape detection from the nurses in the treatment center. She even confided in me about the night she took the overdose.

I did not know how to respond to these psychiatric details, and I did not try. I responded the only way I knew how—I shared. I told her about my struggles with food, my parents, my weight, my shame, and my guilt. She stopped talking and started listening.

I honestly don't know how long we talked. After her explosive venting and my monologue we did actually talk, back and forth, even laughing. We had made the connection. It was a start.

That was fifteen years ago. From those small stuttering steps she has learned to walk. She is now happily married to a devoted husband, has five children whom she schools at home, and she has moved way beyond her bulimia. Her mood and weight are now very stable. She has even reconciled with her parents and is no longer threatened by her twin.

I don't know what I said that made a difference, but I know that it did. Perhaps it was the fact that I just said, I don't know what I would say if it happened again, and it will. I don't know what to tell you except that when you share, you make real contact. And with real contact anything is possible—even change. And every time I make real contact, I become more alive and more invigorated.

Friendship is born at the moment when one person says to another: What you, too! I thought it was only me. – Clive Staples Lewis

Comfort Call—Sandy Warnes

Sandy Warnes describes a moment of reaching out and how comfort, first and foremost, comes primarily from others and only secondarily from food.

I was just about to sit down to dinner when the telephone rang. I thought twice about answering it. It was probably one of those telemarketers, and I wasn't buying. On the other hand it could be a friend in need. I picked it up.

It was one of my weight-loss group buddies. She was struggling. Specifically she was looking at a whole box of cookies and couldn't think of a good reason why she should not eat them. All of them.

For the first minute or so of our conversation, I reiterated the reasons why she should resist the cookie temptation. Any pleasure would be fleeting if she tasted the cookies at all, and she would soon regret her decision. She was doing well and wanted to keep the momentum going. When she got on the scales at the end of the week, she would have long forgotten the temporary comfort that the cookies might now offer.

She listened and agreed, and we quickly moved on to other issues. I asked about her day, and we discussed the trials and tribulations she had experienced. We talked about how she dealt with conflict that had arisen at work and her ensuing anger. She expressed considerable frustration, and I listened. I understood why she was angry and told her that I would have felt the same.

Call friends at times of temptation.

There was a time when I couldn't have helped her. That was when I weighed twice as much as I do now, was irritable, reclusive, and had an inferiority complex the size of an economy-sized zero. I didn't have time for anyone else—I didn't even have time for me. All of that changed nearly ten years ago when I was inspired by seeing a television show that featured Nancy Marasco. Nancy expressed such a positive attitude toward weight loss that day that I was almost instantly motivated to make a serious attempt to lose weight. I joined a group the next week, although, it being Halloween, I did not commit until I could go on and polish off the candy and chocolate to which I was addicted.

I did start attending regularly the week after Halloween, drawn by the non-judgmental warmth and support of the group. Before I realized it I was an active participant, giving as much help as I was getting. I had started to walk with the group members, too. The more I walked with them, the more I cared about them. The more I cared about them, the less insular I became. I didn't realize for quite some time that I had become much more sociable and far less irritable. And thinking about them took the focus off me.

People tell me now that I have "totally changed." It's not just the 120 pounds that I have lost and kept off for over eight years. Not that I am only more sociable now. I act completely differently. Before, the merest criticism would send me into floods of tears; now, I am much stronger and far more assertive. Before, I would barely venture out; now, I give talks in front of hundreds of people. Before, I did not care about other people or about myself. Now, caring for other people is a large part of helping myself.

I have needed my friends along the way. I have needed them for getting me back into the real world and in dealing with the inevitable setbacks, not just of weight loss but also of life. They were there for me, especially a few years ago after I had lost my weight, when I was diagnosed with thyroid cancer. If I needed another reason for being there for them, that was it; but they had already helped me change my life. That's why I picked up the phone—just in case it was one of them.

We talked for about an hour. When the conversation wound down to a natural conclusion, her temptation had gone cold and so had my dinner. The cookies were now irrelevant and offered her nothing. She had gotten her comfort from me rather than from them. We were both happy to be fulfilled rather than just full.

> *The best portion of a man's life, his little, nameless*
> *unremembered acts of kindness and love.*
> *– William Wordsworth*

Rankin's Reminders

Making the Personal Connection

Reach out to others. Extending yourself allows you to help others and hear yourself.

Realize your worth. Your experiences probably seem old and stale to you because you have lived through them, but they are fresh and valuable to others. Your life has worth to other people and thus to you.

Share experiences. Even if the content of your experiences may not mean much to others, your willingness to share them will. It doesn't matter how irrelevant or mundane your experiences may seem, *the act of sharing them* is incredibly powerful.

Step outside yourself. Making a real connection involves temporarily stepping outside your own mental filters and recognizing that there are greater things in the world than your own ego.

Find love through personal relationships, not food. Love comes in many forms and from many different types of people.

Listen. Listen without judgment, and pay full attention. It is amazing what you will find out about the talker and yourself.

Motivate. Actions and words have enormous power. You can motivate and inspire others who have a common goal.

---

[1] A good tactic that in the trade is called **stimulus control**. There is evidence that withdrawal is far worse in situations where the habit has been indulged than in places where it hasn't.

[2] Nicotine does elevate metabolism by up to 10 percent so that when quitting you need fewer calories. However, to compensate for the loss of the oral habit and the return of their taste buds, people frequently eat more. Thus weight gain occurs. In pure health terms, quitting a pack of cigarettes is about the equivalent of losing sixty-five pounds in weight.

[3] You can read Debbee's story on page 194.

Chapter 8

One Hundred Great Weight-Loss Tactics

In the preceding chapters there have been many valuable weight-loss tactics endorsed by people who have lost literally hundreds of pounds and kept them off. Each summary at the end of each chapter has provided a list of seven psychological tips that not only have been proven in use but also by psychological research. In addition, various behavioral tactics endorsed by the contributors to this book have also been highlighted throughout.

Most of the tactics were endorsed by many, if not all, of the successful people featured in this book. It is apparent that attending a weekly group meeting, being aware of food intake—mainly by using a food and exercise journal—drinking at least eight glasses of water a day, measuring portion sizes, participating in a regular exercise program, setting small realistic behavioral goals and weight expectations, and limiting fat intake were almost universally adopted and considered critical to weight-loss success.

Psychologically being accountable for behavior, having support, recognizing responsibility, maintaining an adaptive attitude, making weight loss a priority, visualizing success, keeping in touch with personal motivation, and planning were also essential for success.

So here they are. One hundred psychological and behavioral tactics that will help you achieve your weight-loss goals.

1. **Manage time.** Don't commit your time without thinking about whether this is draining or enhancing.

2. **Know your friends.** Make a list of those who empower you and those who disempower you. Avoid the latter, if possible.

3. **Always sit down to eat.** You're more likely to focus on the food, and thus your overall consumption, if you're not on the run.

4. **Be assertive.** Don't be afraid to say no!

5. **Focus on changing one behavior at a time**. Trying to change several behaviors at once is overwhelming and a set-up for failure.

6. **Determine what situations make you feel helpless**. How can you cope with these better, i.e., other than eating?

7. **Never miss a workout**. Exercise is an appointment with yourself that you have to keep.

8. **Be proactive**. Recognize that difficulty is not the same as helplessness.

9. **Define your boundaries**. Know limits of where and how far others can encroach.

10. **Don't sneak or hide food**. If you're going to eat, eat. If you're ashamed and embarrassed about your eating, don't eat.

11. **Don't sulk or whine**. Self-pity, doubt, and fear will erode your choices.

12. **Find a positive support group**. Your self-esteem can only be improved through positive interaction with others.

13. **Remove yourself from the company of negative, judgmental people**. They will hook your self-doubt and sense of inadequacy and bring you down.

14. **Don't set yourself up for failure**. You are primed to jump to negative conclusions about yourself. Set small, attainable goals, and focus on the short term. Think about losing the next pound, not the next fifty.

15. **Avoid leftovers**. Let others clear the kitchen.

16. **Be aware of those critical internal tapes**. Listen to how you are talking to yourself. Be compassionate with yourself.

17. **Find rewards other than food**. It's good to reward yourself for reaching short-term goals, ideally on a weekly basis. Beauty or health treatments, tickets, CD's, etc., make good rewards.

18. **Eliminate extreme words** like "always" and "never," as well as obligation words like "ought" and "should," from your vocabulary.

19. **Chew sugarless gum to offset hunger**. Chewing gum can also be a great first response to temptation.

20. **Ask yourself: "Am I hungry, or do I want to eat because of some other issue?"**

21. **Find a positive role model.** Imitating success is a great way to achieve it.

22. **Have courage.** Fear is natural but should not stop you.

23. **Walk after meals, especially the evening meal.** Not only will this boost metabolism, but it will also get you away from food at a high temptation time, i.e., just after having eaten.

24. **Don't keep tempting foods around the house if you cannot cope with them.**

25. **Seek professional help if your eating is out of control.** Sometimes it is not possible to overcome the inertia of long-term patterns on your own.

26. **Create a negative-free zone.** Check troubles, anxieties, and doubts at the door, and enjoy a safe haven.

27. **Weigh only once a week.** Weighing more often than this is an unreliable measure of fat loss and is likely to set you up for disappointment.

28. **Have hope.** Your potential is limitless. Reach out, and grab it.

29. **Learn from other people's mistakes.** There's not enough time for you to make them all.

30. **Think movement as well as exercise.** Simply increasing your movement is a great way to start or supplement structured exercise. Walk, stretch, move at every opportunity.

31. **Look on the bright side.** Find the positive aspects in every event. You never really know what an event means at the time it's happening, so make a decision to turn it into a positive.

32. **Measure portions meticulously.** Underestimation of portion size is one of the biggest reasons people don't lose weight.

33. **Don't worry.** Worrying achieves little. Negative energy spent on things that may never happen is a waste.

34. **Eliminate fried food.** Batter is not better.

35. **Eat breakfast.** It is important to give yourself energy at the

beginning of the day to avoid dangerous blood-glucose slumps later. Great meal to get important fruits.

36. **See the humor.** Try to find the funny side. You cannot be miserable while you are laughing.

37. **Don't procrastinate.** Carpe diem—Seize the day!

38. **Use small bowls and plates.** Estimation of food intake is proportional to the size of the plate. The bigger the plate, the more you will eat.

39. **Ensure healthy foods are available at social gatherings.** Bring your own if necessary. You would if it were a matter of life and death—and it is.

40. **Visit a health professional regularly.** Feedback on your health and behavior provides information, motivation, and accountability.

41. **Face fears.** If you can have the courage to face your worst fears, you won't be forever running from them.

42. **Believe in yourself and your ability to lose weight.** Belief is the most important tool you have. Without it, you're lost.

43. **Visualize success.** Images have a powerful effect on the subconscious and the body. If you can't imagine success, you can't achieve it.

44. **Use the Exchange System to guide nutritional choices.**

45. **Don't go shopping for food when you are hungry.**

46. **Maintain positive energy.** Energy translates into a positive mood and positive thoughts. Exercise is the best way of maintaining high energy levels.

47. **Understand which part of you is destructive to health and weight loss.** You have many sides to you. Which parts are healthy and which destructive? Who is doing the destructive eating?

48. **Don't eat anything after 7 P.M.** This helps digestion and metabolism and cuts out evening snacks.

49. **Visualize workouts as a battle against fat.** Strong images can reinforce motivation and help you stay focused.

50. **Take control.** Assert the healthy side of you; control immature, destructive, and helpless feelings.

51. **Be conscious of your binging.** Avoid binge triggers; don't keep binge food at home, and try not to eat alone.

52. **Call friends if you are struggling.** A real connection will make you forget about food.

53. **Drink at least sixty-four ounces of water daily.** Glug it, sip it, slurp it, but get it.

54. **Learn to deal with hunger.** It fades after a while and is manageable.

55. **Remember that your body is your unconscious.** Find peace—meditate, relax, and laugh.

56. **Enlist others to help you start, and then continue, an exercise program.** Accountability and support are everything.

57. **Keep your food chart on your refrigerator.** In sight, in mind.

58. **Indulge in friendly competition.** Find someone with a similar amount of weight to lose.

59. **It's up to you.** Don't imagine anyone or anything else can lose weight or you.

60. **Be informed.** Find out as much as you can about nutrition, exercise, weight loss, and your own body.

61. **Be active in your health care.** Ask questions; do research.

62. **Buy smart.** Invest in products that are aimed at helping you help yourself, not making it sound easy.

63. **Don't make genetics or anything else an excuse.** I'm sorry if you think you have the wrong genes, but that doesn't stop you from taking responsibility for being the healthiest you can be.

64. **Watch your alcohol consumption.** Alcohol is a subtle diet-buster. Willpower dissolves in alcohol.

65. **Avoid high-risk situations.** Don't put yourself in harm's way unless you really have to.

66. **Don't be afraid of hard work.** Lifestyle change is not for wimps.

67. **Put down the gun.** There's no magic bullet.

68. **Make the decision.** Anything is possible once you have decided to do it.

69. **Keep food scales in the kitchen easily available.** It's easy to become complacent, not weigh or measure, and completely underestimate your food intake.

70. **Go public.** Tell as many people as possible about your goals.

71. **Read nutrition labels.** Pay special attention to the serving size of the product—the information can be misleading, especially on small packages that you assume are one serving size but are not listed as such.

72. **Define your goals.** Be specific. Make goals tangible, behavioral targets (e.g., I'm not going to eat more than thirty grams of fat a day) rather than vague ideas (I'm going to lose ten pounds).

73. **Regularly review your behavior.** Eliminate routines and habits that have outlived their usefulness.

74. **Eat favorite foods in moderation.** You can learn that you only need a taste.

75. **Set manageable weekly weight goals.** Set a realistic weight loss for the upcoming week.

76. **Be prepared.** Take healthy snacks like fruit, pretzels, and yogurt with you so that there is always a healthy alternative.

77. **Write a contract.** Write a contract that specifies what behaviors you are going to change.

78. **Find good ways of dealing with fatigue.** Drink water; take a nap; avoid sugar.

79. **Don't believe weight-loss stories and claims that are too good to be true.** They generally are false and set up unrealistic expectations.

80. **Make it a priority.** Write exercise times in your diary, and keep them as sacred appointments. Whatever else happens, ensure you meet your goal for the day.

81. **Learn how to refuse food.** It's not only okay; it's essential to not be swayed by the guilt trips and agendas of others.

82. **Stay connected to your motivation.** Remember the pain that made you want to lose weight in the first place.

83. **Reach out to others.** Extending yourself allows you to help them and heal yourself.

84. **Realize your worth.** Your experiences probably seem old and stale to you because you have lived through them, but they are fresh and valuable to others. Your life has worth to other people and thus to you.

85. **Savor food.** Eat slowly, and enjoy the tastes and textures of food.

86. **Increase exercise when you hit a weight plateau.** When you get stuck, give your metabolism an extra kick by increasing your exercise.

87. **Don't eat other people's food.** Don't take food off other plates.

88. **Share experiences.** Even if the content of your experiences may not mean much to others, your willingness to share them will. It doesn't matter how irrelevant or mundane your experiences may seem, *the act of sharing them* is incredibly powerful.

89. **Eat away from stress, noise, and chaos.** Stress will only increase the speed of eating and thus your intake. It will also give you heartburn.

90. **Eliminate sodas.** Water is the best choice.

91. **Visualize being successful.** See yourself thinner, making the right choices, exercising. Rehearse this image on a daily basis.

92. **Step outside yourself.** Making a real connection involves temporarily stepping outside your own mental filters and recognizing that there are greater things in the world than your own ego.

93. **Find love through personal relationships, not food.** Love comes in many forms and from many different types of people.

94. **Listen.** Listen without judgment, and pay full attention. It is amazing what you will discover about the talker and yourself.

95. **Switch from dairy desserts to yogurt.** Similar taste, big calorie difference.

96. **Motivate.** Actions and words have enormous power. You can motivate and inspire others who have a common goal.

97. **Minimize salad dressing.** Salad dressing is typically high calorie. Go for diet dressings on the side.

98. **Exercise patience with yourself and with others.** You can't do it all at once. Good things take time.

99. **Ask yourself: "Is this food (or action) getting me nearer my**

Howard J. Rankin, Ph.D

As the nationally acclaimed author of 7 Steps to Wellness, 10 Steps to a Great Relationship, and Power Talk: The Art of Effective Communication, Howard J. Rankin is in demand whenever and wherever people want to learn about how to take charge of their health and their lives.

Howard's goal in both his writing and his highly celebrated seminar series is to provide practical tools for overcoming life's obstacles. Through his research, academic background, and vast clinical experience, Howard teaches people to motivate, communicate, and develop resilience. He is just as effective in large organizations as he is with small groups.

Howard is as comfortable doing stand-up comedy as he is when delivering a serious keynote address. Using previous experiences as a comedy writer, and as the only person ever to have written a scientific paper in limerick form, Rankin is an entertaining as well as inspirational speaker. He has a natural ability to turn academic and research data into easily understood principles with real-life application. As a result his seminars are highly acclaimed. Howard has been described as "the best stand-up comedian in the serious subject of health," "a master communicator," and "the leading lifestyle change expert."

Howard's work has been featured on ABC's *20/20*, as well as on CNN and other national television and radio shows. He has been a consultant to the World Health Organization and the National Institute on Drug Abuse. Howard's work has also been featured in many newspapers and print media including *The Wall Street Journal, The Los Angeles Times, The Baltimore Sun, The Dallas Morning News, The Cleveland Plain Dealer, Ladies Home Journal, Prevention, Family Circle, Mademoiselle, Health, New Woman,* and *Weight Watchers,* to name but a few.

Seminars

Inspirational, humorous, and practical — these are the hallmarks of Howard's seminars, keynotes, and workshops. Howard has delivered hundreds of talks over the years. Here are some of his favorites.

Stop Talking, Start Communicating highlights the fundamental principles of communication, as outlined in Howard's book, *Power Talk: The Art of Effective Communication*. This seminar teaches not just effective listening but also verbal and nonverbal techniques that will motivate and inspire others. Enjoyed by executives, sales people, parents, teachers, couples—anyone who wants to have more influence in the world.

Resilience is not your typical stress-management talk. Drawing on his work in stress, trauma, and inspirational stories of change, Howard outlines then teaches the fundamentals of coping. A powerful presentation that will inoculate you against life's troubles.

Your Body Is Your Subconscious goes way beyond yoga and meditation. Howard delivers crucial evidence of the mind-body connection and shows how anyone can take advantage of this emerging field. Learn how such concepts as hope, responsibility, and control can affect the molecules in your body and how language and imagery could save your life.

In **Where's My Motivation Gone?** Howard shows why motivation ebbs and flows and how you can develop it and keep it in the forefront of your mind. Using his *motivational link method*, Howard teaches techniques that develop and maintain drive to help you realize your goals and dreams.

From Dr. Howard J. Rankin

7 Steps to Wellness

This book shows you how to control your weight and your life! Most people know what they need to do to lose weight, manage stress, and stay in shape, but doing it is another matter. Dr. Howard Rankin shows 7 Steps that you need to take for optimal health and performance.

Learn how to …

Capture motivation—and maintain it.

Develop self-management skills.

Develop positive thinking.

Develop self-control.

Defeat binging.

Cope with high risks.

Get the support you want.

Comes with nutrition and exercise guide, fourteen-day meal plan, daily journal, and eating-out guide.

NEWLY REVISED!

ISBN 0-9658261-1-2   **Price $12.95**

Published by Stepwise Press. Available at booksellers, on the web at www.findpeace.com, or by calling (843) 842-7797.

10 Steps to a Great Relationship

What every couple should know about love ...

Dr. Howard Rankin explores the secrets of a great relationship and describes ten steps that make real love.

Discover ...

The dynamics of attraction.

The five stages of a relationship.

How to keep romance alive.

Ten rules of fighting fair.

The secrets of intimacy.

How to communicate more effectively.

How to keep your independence in a relationship.

How, when, and why to practice forgiveness.

And much more!

NEWLY REVISED!

ISBN 0-9658261-2-0   **Price $12.95**

Published by Stepwise Press. Available at booksellers, on the web at www.findpeace.com, or by calling (843) 842-7797.

Power Talk: The Art of Effective Communication

Good communication is motivation. Whether you are a CEO, a teacher, a doctor, an executive, a salesperson, a coach, or a parent, this book shows you how to develop relationships and motivate with power.

Combining the best social-science research, neuro-linguistic programming, and experience gained in a long career as a psychotherapist, Dr. Howard Rankin shows how you can improve your communication and your influence.

Discover ...

How to create powerful messages that work.

Why "the experience is the message."

Seven Fundamental Motivators.

How to overcome resistance.

The where, why, and how of listening.

Secrets of hypnotic language patterns.

The power of stories, metaphors, and humor.

How to develop instant rapport.

ISBN 0-9658261-3-9   **Price $11.95**

Published by Stepwise Press. Available at booksellers, on the web at www.findpeace.com, or by calling (843) 842-7797.

TOPS

TOPS Club, Inc., is the oldest nonprofit, noncommercial, weight-loss support group and has over 235,000 members worldwide. Mrs. Esther Manz founded TOPS in 1948.

Members lose weight sensibly through a combination of healthful dieting, exercise, setting realistic goals, and the group support of TOPS. Since 1966 TOPS Club, Inc., has donated over $5.4 million toward obesity research.

There are various ways to contact the Take Off Pounds Sensibly Club, Inc. You can call 1-800-932-8677 for the location of the nearest TOPS chapter and a free brochure about taking off pounds sensibly.

You can also visit the TOPS website—www.tops.org—where you can find information about local meetings, as well as the latest news about the organization, its members, and current articles on weight loss and health.

You can write to TOPS Club, Inc., 4575 Fifth St., Milwaukee, Wisconsin 53207-5800.